THE

VITAMIN

C

CONTROVERSY:

QUESTIONS

AND

ANSWERS

by

Emanuel Cheraskin, M.D., D.M.D.

Bio-Communications Press
3100 North Hillside Avenue
Wichita, Kansas 67219

BIO-COMMUNICATIONS PRESS
3100 North Hillside Avenue
Wichita, Kansas 67219 USA

ISBN 0-942333-01-2
Library of Congress Catalog Card Number: 87-71003

First Edition

Published in The United States of America

The information on vitamin C contained in this book has
been compiled from a variety of sources and is subject to
differences of opinion and interpretation. This book is not
intended as a source of medical advice, and any questions
on individual use of vitamin C, general or specific, should
be addressed to the reader's nutrition-oriented physician.

BCP and Bio-Communications Press are service marks of The Olive
W. Garvey Center for the Improvement of Human Functioning, Inc.

It's not what he doesn't know that bothers me,
it's what he knows for sure that just ain't so.

Will Rogers

TABLE OF CONTENTS

Acknowledgements xiii

Preface: Why This Monograph? xv

Introduction xvi

Part One The Epidemiology of Vitamin C

1. How Prevalent is Hypovitaminosis C in Population Groups? 3

2. How Big a Problem is Suboptimal Vitamin C Tissue State in Ordinary Working People? 5

3. How Common is a Vitamin C Deficiency in a Dental School Patient Population? 7

4. What is the Daily Dietary Vitamin C Consumption of Dentists? 9

5. How Big a Problem is Vitamin C Tissue Deficiency in Orthodontic Patients? 11

6. What is the Vitamin C Health of Dental Students? 13

Part Two The Measurement of Vitamin C

7. What is the Present Most Common Way of Biochemically Establishing Vitamin C State? 17

8. What is the Intradermal Ascorbic Acid Test? 19

9. What is the Lingual Vitamin C Test? 21

10. How Does Plasma Ascorbic Acid Correlate with the Lingual Vitamin C Test? 23

viii

11. How Significant is the Relationship Between Dietary Vitamin C Consumption and Vitamin C Tissue State as Judged by Measurement in the Tongue?   27

12. How do the Skin and Tongue Vitamin C Diagnostic Tests Compare?   29

13. How Sensitive is Vitamin C Nutriture to Dietary Intake?   33

Part Three   Vitamin C in General Health and Disease

14. Are There Overall Known Correlations Between Vitamin C and General Health?   39

15. What About Vitamin C Consumption and Respiratory Findings?   43

16. Can One Identify Any Possible Connection Between Vitamin C and Cardiovascular Symptomatology?   47

17. Vitamin C Consumption and Fatigability?   51

18. Is There Any Possible Connection Between Vitamin C and the Skin?   53

19. Are There Known Relationships Between Vitamin C and the Electrocardiogram?   57

20. Can Contact Lens Intolerance be Altered with Vitamin C Intake?   61

21. Is the Relationship of Chronologic to Bone Age in Any Way Dependent upon Vitamin C?   63

22. Time Release—A Helpful Adjunct?   67

Part Four   Vitamin C in Oral Health and Disease

23. Can One Demonstrate Changes in Gingival Hue by Means of Simple Orange Juice Supplementation?   75

24. What About Vitamin C and Subclinical Scurvy?   77

25. Is There Any Correlation Between Blood and/or Tissue Vitamin C State and Clinical Tooth Mobility?   79

26. Can One Relate Blood Ascorbic Acid Levels to Sulcus Depth?   83

27. Can One Connect Tissue Vitamin C State to Sulcus Depth?   85

28. Of What Possible Importance Might Vitamin C be in Alveolar Bone Loss?   87

29. What About a Connection Between Oral Hygiene and Vitamin C Tissue State?   95

30. What About a Possible Relationship Between Blood Vitamin C and Oral Hygiene?   99

31. Is There a Known Connection Between Oral Tartar (Calculus) and Tissue Vitamin C State?   103

32. What Demonstrated Connection Can One Show Between Tartar on the Teeth and Blood Vitamin C Level?   107

33. Is Oral Hygiene (However Defined) Related to Vitamin C State?   109

34. Are There Any Advantages in Utilizing Sustained-Release Multivitamins Including Vitamin C for the Treatment of Gingival Pathology?   113

x

35. Is There Any Justification for Time-Release
     Vitamin Supplementation in Oral Health?   115

36. Vitamin C and the Water Soluble
     Bioflavonoids—Are They Synergistic:
     A Study of Clinical Tooth Mobility?   117

Part Five   Diet and Vitamin C State

37. What About the Effect of Dietary Vitamin C
     upon Vitamin C State?   123

38. Can Protein Supplementation Influence the
     Vitamin C State?   129

39. What About Sugar and Vitamin C State?   133

Part Six   Vitamin C and Metabolism

40. Is There Any Possible Relationship Between
     Serum Cholesterol and Vitamin C State?   137

41. Is There Any Correlation Between Vitamin
     C Levels Under Tolerance Conditions
     in Smokers Versus Nonsmokers?   141

42. What if Any is the Relationship Between Car-
     bohydrate Metabolism and Vitamin C State?   145

43. What Happens to Vitamin C Tissue Levels
     Following a Three-Day Multivitamin/Trace
     Mineral Versus Placebo Supplement?   151

**Part Seven   Vitamin C as a Predictive
                Instrument**

44. Can One Utilize Vitamin C Tissue Status as a
     Predictor of Gingival Response to the Clean-
     ing and Polishing of the Teeth?   157

45. Are There Other Evidences of the Use of
Vitamin C as a Predictor of Oral Response to
Local Therapy?   159

Part Eight   The "Ideal" Vitamin C State

46. Is it Possible to Establish an "Ideal" Daily
Vitamin C Intake?   163

47. What is the "Ideal" Intradermal Ascorbic Acid
Test Range?   167

48. Do High and Low Vitamin C Users Differ in
Other Dietary Habits?   171

49. What do We Know About Human Vitamin C
Requirements?   173

50. What Can We Say About the "Ideal" Lingual
Vitamin C Test Score Range?   177

Appendix   181

Index   195

ACKNOWLEDGMENTS

Clearly, a production of this kind is never a one-man job. I have had help. Wonderful assistance from many sources. First, grateful acknowledgment is made to the many journals and publishers who originally released these experimental reports. There are too many to acknowledge here. However, they are all listed in the Appendix.

The hard work, the on-hands contributions have been accomplished by Sara Gay at the University of Alabama Medical Center along with Barbara Nichols, Donna Schrag and Jill McKown at The Olive W. Garvey Center for the Improvement of Human Functioning.

Finally, my grateful appreciation to Hugh D. Riordan, M.D., President of The Olive W. Garvey Center for the insight which led to the genesis of Bio-Communications Press. Obviously, without his understanding and efforts, this monograph would never have been possible.

Emanuel Cheraskin, M.D., D.M.D.

PREFACE: WHY THIS MONOGRAPH?

Four reasons.

First, since the advent of Linus Pauling's book **Vitamin C and the Common Cold** in 1970, there has been a renaissance of interest (with its attendant debate) about the role of ascorbic acid in health and disease.

Secondly, quite apart from this movement, my colleagues and I, over the past thirty years, have shared in approximately 1000 clinical experiments eventuating in about 80 published papers in the technical literature (which are listed in chronologic order at the end of this manuscript).

Thirdly, while much of our clinical investigations have resulted in areas of interest to ourselves as well as others, we would like to think that some of our efforts have been truly singular. Three quick examples—our interest in testing for vitamin C by unique methodology, namely in the skin and tongue, our concern with vitamin C and stomatology and finally, the not-often-discussed business of normal ("healthy") versus normal ("average").

Fourth and lastly, during these many years, we have been asked (increasingly with the burgeoning interest) many good questions from many different and diverse people about vitamin C in general to which we have responded with a book entitled **The Vitamin C Connection** (see Appendix). We have also been queried on many occasions regarding our own work. Accordingly, this monograph has included the answers to the fifty most commonly requested answers to studies done in our own laboratory.

Emanuel Cheraskin, M.D., D.M.D.

INTRODUCTION

Knowing more about vitamin C and how it affects our lives, health and energy is probably one of the most important pieces of information we can have to reduce the likelihood of getting disease or becoming dis-eased.

As one of the few animal species on earth incapable of making its own vitamin C, humans need to fully appreciate the importance of obtaining optimal amounts of this essential nutrient.

While every standard medical textbook cites the many problems associated with too little vitamin C, very few physicians ever do the relatively simple tests which determine how much vitamin C their patients have in their blood, urine and tissues.

Increasingly, researchers are discovering what Mother Nature has known and implemented to allow humans to survive as well as they have. Mother Nature knew to make breast milk rich in vitamin C and to create the mechanism which allows the anterior chamber of the eye to have six times the vitamin C level of the plasma which brings the nutrient to the eye.

By reading this book each person concerned with the health of others and with their own health will learn a body of knowledge which is enormously important to the successful building and maintaining of the human immune system.

Hugh D. Riordan, M.D.

PART

ONE

THE

EPIDEMIOLOGY

OF

VITAMIN

C

If we exclude straightforward famine, scurvy is probably the nutritional deficiency disease that has caused most suffering in recorded history.

Kenneth J. Carpenter
The History of Scurvy
and Vitamin C 1986

1. How Prevalent is Hypovitaminosis C in Population Groups?

A fascinating report entitled **Adult Scurvy** appeared in 1985 in the Journal of the American Medical Association in which the authors point out the protean nature of adult scurvy and raise the burning question as to the real incidence and prevalence of vitamin C deficiency.

In this connection, we responded with an article entitled "The Prevalence of Hypovitaminosis C" in the Journal of the American Medical Association (254: #20, 2894, 22/29 November 1985) by pointing out that Schorah, who is fully cited in that report, reviewed the literature on this very subject. He concluded (Table 1.1) that some-

Table 1.1

proportion of population groups
with low leukocyte vitamin C reserves
(approximate values)

group	A*	B**
young, healthy	3	0
elderly, healthy	20	3
elderly, outpatients	68	20
patients with cancer	76	46
institutionalized elderly	95	50
institutionalized young	100	30

* A indicates percentage of subjects with marginal vitamin C deficiency state.
** B indicates percentage of subjects with classical scurvy.

where between 3 percent of young and healthy subjects and 100 percent of institutionalized young suffer from marginal hypovitaminosis C and 0 percent (healthy young subjects) to 50 percent (institutionalized elderly) may possibly demonstrate full-blown classical scurvy.

These points are emphasized in Table 1.1. Column A

indicates the figures for subclinical vitamin C deficiency; Column B, those who could be deemed as suffering from obvious classical scurvy.

We have been studying this problem in our clinic at the University of Alabama Medical Center for a number of years in five unique populations with over 4000 subjects including: (1) a dental school patient population, (2) patients in a dental prepayment program, (3) orthodontic patients, (4) selected groups of Floridian dentists and their staffs and (5) dental students. Depending upon the tests and the standards for normality (and these topics are discussed in Part Two, The Measurement of Vitamin C), we have concluded that somewhere between 17 percent and 72 percent of the subjects studied by us demonstrated suboptimal to clearcut ascorbic acid deficiency levels.

If indeed the figures summarized by Schorah and those cited by us reflect the true epidemiologic status of ascorbic acid deficiency, then hypovitaminosis C is a very real and common, probably epidemic, problem which clearly has not been properly viewed and surely not adequately reported.

2. How Big a Problem is Suboptimal Vitamin C Tissue State in Ordinary Working People?

The nonfasting lingual vitamin C test scores (and this procedure is spelled out in Question 9 beginning on page 21) were determined in 1305 employees in the culinary industry and 762 child dependents of employees in the retail clerks industry. This makes for a total of 2067 subjects who participated in this experiment (Table 2.1). The workers in the culinary industry included cooks, waiters, waitresses, and bartenders. The 762 children were dependents of the members of Retail Clerks Local 770 in Los Angeles. All of these observations were reported in an article entitled "A Lingual Vitamin C Test: VIII. Vitamin C State in a Dental Prepayment Program" which we published in the International Journal for Vitamin Research (38: #3/4, 421-423, 1968).

The accompanying chart (Table 2.1) summarizes the

Table 2.1

lingual vitamin C scores

nonfasting lingual time groups (seconds)	number and percentage of subjects		
	culinary workers	dependents of retail clerks	total
0-19	361 (27.7%)	225 (29.5%)	586 (28.4%)
20-39	743 (56.9%)	311 (40.8%)	1054 (51.0%)
40+	201 (15.4%)	226 (29.7%)	427 (20.7%)
totals	1305(100.0%)	762(100.0%)	2067(100.0%)*
mean	27.6	31.4	29.0
standard deviation	12.7	15.7	14.0

* approximate

results. It will be noted that, for the entire sample, the mean and standard deviation is 29.0 ± 14.0 seconds. Thus, two-thirds of the sample ranges from 15 to 43 seconds. The majority of subjects (51 percent) showed lingual times of approximately 20 to 39 seconds. The rest of the scores were almost equally dispersed between short times (0 to 19 seconds) and relatively long times (40+ seconds).

Utilizing a physiologic standard of less than 20 seconds (and this matter is discussed in Part Eight The "Ideal" Vitamin C State), 51 percent of the group showed scores which can be regarded as marginally suboptimal and 21 percent of the sample displayed values consistent with an obvious and frank ascorbic acid deficiency.

The point which should be underlined is that, within the limits of this simple study of middle class people in California, it is safe to say that a significant percentage, actually a majority, might well be suffering with a vitamin C deficiency state and, according to some investigators, the scope of the problem is, therefore, of truly epidemic and serious proportions.

3. How Common is a Vitamin C Deficiency in a Dental School Patient Population?

There is surprisingly little in the literature regarding the incidence and prevalence of vitamin C deficiency in the total population. Hence, it is not surprising that there is little offered in connection with the scope of the problem in subsets of our population including patients who visit a dental school for mouth care.

The answer to this question was made possible from a study of 861 routine oral care subjects who were examined in the Department of Oral Medicine at the University of Alabama School of Dentistry. This was subsequently reported in an article entitled "Vitamin C State in a Dental School Patient Population" in the Journal of the Southern California State Dental Association (32: #10, 375-378, October 1964).

It is important to underline that vitamin C state was judged by three different techniques. Firstly, it was measured in blood. Specifically, ascorbic acid levels were ascertained for the entire sample of 861 subjects (271 in the fasting state; and 590 nonfasting or two-hour postprandial). Particulars regarding this type of vitamin C measurement is provided in Question 7 which begins on page 17. It was recognized at that time that, in the opinion of many authorities, plasma levels were then and still are viewed as more a function of dietary intake than tissue concentration. Accordingly, two other techniques were employed. The vitamin C state was estimated by the intradermal technique in 560 of the 861 participants. A description of this method of ascertaining tissue vitamin C concentration is described in Question 8 beginning on page 19. Actually, 221 determinations were made under fasting conditions and 339 two-hours postprandially. The reason for utilizing only 560 of the 861 subjects was due to the fact that, as a dermal colorization test, it can only be performed on caucasian subjects. Notwithstanding, it is, as far as we can determine, the only such study of vitamin

C state in this particular tissue. Finally, the lingual decolorization technique was employed in 229 subjects (102 fasting; 127 nonfasting). This very interesting method for ascertaining tissue levels is considered in Question 9 beginning on page 21. The reason for the relatively small sample by the latter method was due to the fact that this test had been introduced late in the survey. Parenthetic mention should be made that this is the only tissue determination of vitamin C ever recorded in the epidemiologic literature.

It is difficult to estimate the extent of vitamin C deficiency by these three methods since there is relatively little agreement as to the physiologic range by any of the presenting testing techniques. This subject will be dealt with elsewhere in this monograph. For more discussion, please refer to Part Eight The "Ideal" Vitamin C State.

However, to the extent that one can draw a conclusion, the evidence suggests, at a minimum, that as much as one-half of the studied sample demonstrates a vitamin C level indicative of a possible marginal ascorbic acid deficiency state.

Most importantly, it would seem that the prime point of this story is that, by whatever methodology, there seems to be reasonable evidence that vitamin C deficiency is common and may indeed be a pandemic problem.

4. What is the Daily Dietary Vitamin C Consumption of Dentists?

There are several ways of looking at the epidemiology of vitamin C deficiency. One is to examine the biochemical aspects of the problem. A second approach is to look at dietary habits. We thought it might be of interest to report the daily ascorbic acid consumption of 1086 dentists and their spouses whom we had examined over a four-year period in a multiple health testing program. It is well to add that these subjects were considered to be of above-average health on the basis of an examination, namely a self-administered health questionnaire and an indepth analysis of blood and urine along with dietary inquiry.

Parenthetic mention should be made that both the American Medical Association and the American Dental Association have noted that participants in health screening programs are usually more health conscious than the average doctor and his spouse.

Table 4.1
distribution of daily vitamin C consumption
(seven-day diet diary)

mg. vitamin C daily	number of subjects	percentage of subjects
0- 60	136	12.5
61-120	373	34.3
121-180	323	29.8
181-240	158	14.6
241+	96	8.8
total	1086	100.0
mean	140.3	
standard deviation	80.5	
minimum	4	
maximum	666	

From a seven-day dietary diary, the daily vitamin C consumption expressed in milligrams was calculated from food tables prepared by the United States Department of Agriculture. We put this information together from the doctors and their families and published the results in an article entitled "Dentists Need More Vitamin

10

C?" which we released in the Journal of the Tennessee Dental Association (57: #4, 177-178, October 1977).

Utilizing a 60 mg. per day recommended dietary allowance (RDA) for vitamin C which had been established in 1968, 136 subjects, namely 12.5 percent, were not meeting this requirement (Table 4.1). In other words, approximately one out of eight dentists and their spouses were subsisting on a suboptimal vitamin C regime. It should be pointed out that, in 1973 the Food and Nutrition Board revised the RDA for vitamin C to 45 mg. per day (Table 4.2). Utilizing this new index of dietary vitamin C adequacy, 74 subjects (6.8 percent) were found to be subsisting on an inadequate regime.

Table 4.2

distribution of daily vitamin C
consumption
(seven-day diet diary)

mg. vitamin C daily	number of subjects	percentage of subjects
0- 44	74	6.8
45- 90	220	20.3
91- 180	537	49.4
181- 269	189	17.4
250+	66	6.1
total	1086	100.0
mean	140.3	
standard deviation	80.5	
minimum	4	
maximum	666	

Since doctors and their spouses, as has already been indicated, who participate in such studies are usually more health conscious and above average in health status, one can only speculate as to how many doctors and their families fit the category for suboptimal deficiency. Additionally, if interferences in the metabolism of vitamin C are also included, clearly the percentage with marginal vitamin C nutriture increases. For example, it is well known that smoking decreases the intestinal absorption of vitamin C and approximately 12 percent of these doctors and their spouses smoked 10 or more cigarettes per day.

In any case, however, these data are viewed, they strongly suggest that a significant segment of the dental professional population is subsisting on a suboptimal vitamin C regime.

5. How Big a Problem is Vitamin C Tissue Deficiency in Orthodontic Patients?

There is no question but that the orthodontic experience involves the deliberate destruction of bone in certain areas (with the hope that bone elsewhere will be reformed). Clearly, this is the basis for tooth movement. Additionally, there is no argument but that vitamin C is an essential ingredient in the deposition of osteoid matrix which, in turn, is required for new bone formation.

For these and other reasons, we were curious to try to establish the extent of suboptimal vitamin C deficiency state in routine orthodontic patients.

Accordingly, this was a study of the ascorbic acid state (as measured by the lingual vitamin C test technique) in 139 routine orthodontic patients. We subsequently reported this information in a paper entitled "Biology of the Orthodontic Patient: II. Lingual Vitamin C Test Scores" which we published in the Angle Orthodontist (39: #4, 324-325, October 1969).

Table 5.1

lingual vitamin C test scores distribution

lingual vitamin C scores (seconds)	number and percentage of subjects
10-14	5 (3.6%)
15-19	34 (24.5%)
20-24	25 (18.0%)
25-29	32 (23.0%)
30-34	15 (10.8%)
35-39	12 (9.8%)
40-44	7 (5.0%)
45-49	2 (1.4%)
50-60	7 (5.0%)
total	139 (100.0%)*

* approximate

According to the best available evidence, the physiologic range for the lingual vitamin C test is approximately 15 to 20 seconds. This matter is discussed elsewhere in greater detail. Table 5.1 shows the number and percentage of subjects according to lingual vitamin C test grades.

On this basis, approximately 72 percent of the subjects display suboptimal ascorbic acid tissue state.

It is, therefore, of interest that approximately, by this method, 7 out of 10 orthodontic patients show vitamin C scores which are marginal if not definitely poor.

Additional articles have resulted from our observations of the relationship between vitamin C and the orthodontic patient. These are listed in the Appendix. For the moment, the evidence is also clear that vitamin C nutriture as measured by plasma ascorbic acid levels also demonstrates that vitamin C nutrition is very poor in subjects undergoing orthodontic treatment.

6.   What is the Vitamin C Health of Dental Students?

The complete study consisted of performing plasma ascorbic acid levels and intradermal times simultaneously in forty-two presumably healthy and young dental students. The determinations were made regularly at 10:00 A.M. when the students arrived for their clinic duties. The subjects were not informed that these tests would be done. Consequently, there were no preparatory instructions. However, at the time these tests were done, histories of citrus consumption and tobacco habits were recorded because it is well known of the role of citrus intake in the overall ascorbic acid status of the body and because there are reports in the literature suggesting that smoking alters the level of vitamin C.

For more particulars regarding the latter problem, the reader is referred to Part Six dealing with Vitamin C and Metabolism and specifically Question 41 which asks "Is There Any Correlation Between Vitamin C Levels Under Tolerance Conditions in Smokers Versus Nonsmokers?"

Laboratory procedures included plasma ascorbic acid levels and intradermal decolorization times. These were fully described in a subsequent publication entitled "The Intradermal Ascorbic Acid Test: Part III. A Study of Forty-Two Dental Students" which appeared in the Journal of Dental Medicine (13: #3, 135-155, July 1958).

An attempt was made to answer several questions. Specifically, what are the plasma ascorbic acid values of a group of young and presumably healthy dental students? Without delving into all the details, it is clear that the levels ranged from 0.07 to 1.48 mg. percent with a group mean of 0.56 ± 0.36 mg. percent. This means that approximately two-thirds of the subjects varied from 0.29 to 1.01 mg. percent. A rather large standard deviation (0.35 mg. percent) indicates the great degree of individual variation. More pertinent at this point is the fact that there was an almost even distribution of values above and below 0.60 mg. percent. Specifically, 53 percent of the students yielded plasma ascorbic acid levels below

14

0.60 mg. percent. Suffice it to say here that many authorities regard 0.60 mg. percent as the dividing line between normal and subnormal levels. If one accepts this demarcation, then over half of the dental students demonstrated inadequate plasma ascorbic acid levels.

Viewing vitamin C state as judged by tissue concentration (measured in the skin), the values range from 12 to 49 minutes. The mean for this group was 27 minutes with a standard deviation of 9.7 minutes. In other words, approximately two-thirds of the subjects demonstrated intradermal values between 17.3 and 36.7 minutes. There was slightly less individual variation here than apparent from the plasma ascorbic acid values.

Since the intradermal test had not been widely studied and, more important, less accepted than the plasma determinations, there has resulted no intradermal time range with which to gauge health and deficiency with respect to vitamin C. We have tried to solve this problem in Question 47. For the moment, therefore, the mean value of 27 minutes was chosen arbitrarily as a base from which to describe the relative dispersion of scores. The distribution of values on both sides of the mean was about even, namely 52 percent of the subjects revealed disappearance times below 27 minutes.

Judging from the literature, the evidence suggests that the ideal decolorization time is probably 10 to 15 minutes. Hence, one can conclude that, tissuewise, these dental students demonstrate marginal vitamin C state.

In short, the evidence, while certainly not complete, supports the notion that vitamin C status is poor in third-year (junior) dental students.

PART

TWO

THE

MEASUREMENT

OF

VITAMIN

C

The things I can measure I can understand; and those things I cannot measure I cannot understand.

Lord Kelvin

7. What is the Present Most Common Way of Biochemically Establishing Vitamin C State?

The techniques for biochemical evaluation seem today to be at a high point as judged by the number of different biochemical measures and techniques available for the detection, therapeutic appraisal, and prediction of

Table 7.1

plasma ascorbic acid findings from a survey of the literature

author(s)	plasma range (mgm.%)	average (mgm.%)	number of subjects	health
Greenberg, et al. (1936)	.25-1.48	.72	55	medical students
Abt, et al. (1936)	.72-1.32	1.24	54	normal
Ingalls (1937)	.45-1.32	1.00	9	normal
Pijoan and Klemperer (1937)	.65-2.00	?	150	normal
Portnoy and Wilkinson (1938)	.60-1.85	1.25	26	normal
Poncher and Stubenrauch (1938)	.80-1.80	1.01	35	normal
Baksh, et al. (1940)	.30-2.00	1.19	140	normal
Todhunter, et al. (1942)	.84-1.46	1.13	35 tests, 5 subjects	normal
Donelson, et al. (1945)	?	.66	582	college women
Lubschez (1945)	.20-1.60	about .90	63	normal
Roe, et al. (1947)	.05-1.60		50	normal
Kruse (1942)	0-1.40	?	49	normal
Dallyn and Moshette (1952)	.1-2.40	.70±.15	447	grade school children
Roderuck, et al. (1956) boys	.13-2.18	.78		school children,
girls	.12-2.50	.81	655	6-18 yrs.
Banerjee and Belarady (1953)	?	.88±.03	21	normal
Lu, et al. (1957)	.07-1.16	.24±.137	25	normal females
Bonomolo, et al. (1956)	males ?	.75	103	healthy
	females?	.78	75	children
Cheraskin, et al. (1958)	.07-1.48	.65±.36	42	dental students

different and diverse disease states. Some of these biochemical measures are very popular such as blood glucose in the study of diabetes mellitus and serum cholesterol and some of its derivatives in cardiovascular pathosis. In this sense, it is noteworthy that measurements of vitamin C state are rarely employed. When they are used, the plasma ascorbic acid concentration is the most popular measuring approach.

At the time that we became interested in studying the measurement of vitamin C, we naturally reviewed the literature and summarized the material. This led us to believe that the technique of Mindlin and Butler, published in an article entitled "The Determination of Ascorbic Acid in Plasma: A Macromethod and a Micromethod" which appeared in the Journal of Biological Chemistry (122: #3, 673-686, February 1938), was preferred.

Several points became very obvious at that time and, as far as we can determine, still prevail. First of all, actually very few studies have been done to establish a "normal" or "healthy" or "optimal" level of vitamin C in the blood. Table 7.1 summarizes the data at the time that we became involved in measuring vitamin C. We reported our work with plasma ascorbic acid levels in a paper described as "The Intradermal Ascorbic Acid Test: Part III. A Study of Forty-Two Dental Students" which appeared in the Journal of Dental Medicine (13: #3, 135-155, July 1958).

It is noteworthy from Table 7.1 that there are several investigators who have looked at the problem. It is also clear that most of the work was done in the thirties, forties and fifties. In other words, we now have assumed that the final answer has been written or is unimportant as to what the plasma ascorbic level of vitamin C should or could be. Additionally, Table 7.1 underlines the fact that the samples utilized to identify a reasonable range were derived very loosely from samples assumed to be from the healthy population.

For the moment, and this should be borne in mind throughout this monograph, we have extensively used plasma as a measure for vitamin C. The so-called "ideal" levels are discussed in the last section of this monograph. Additionally, on several occasions, we have taken the opportunity of equating plasma ascorbic acid levels versus vitamin C concentration in tissues and notably in the skin and in the tongue.

8.   What is the Intradermal Ascorbic Acid Test?

It is generally agreed among investigators in this area that the blood vitamin C level, and this usually means plasma concentration, appears to be more a measure of dietary intake than tissue saturation. Thus, it is not surprising that there have been numerous attempts to develop other and, hopefully, more adequate testing procedures.

In one of these areas, we have been particularly concerned for a number of years. An examination of the Appendix underscores our interests and efforts in developing tests of the vitamin C state in the skin.

The so-called intradermal ascorbic acid test was originally developed in the 1930s. An extensive analysis of its history and findings have been outlined by us in a paper entitled "The Intradermal Ascorbic Acid Test: Part III. A Study of Forty-Two Dental Students" which was published in the Journal of Dental Medicine (13: #3, 135-155, July 1958).

The skin test was originally designed to ascertain in a quick and relatively simple fashion a reasonable measure of vitamin C state in the integument.

Because the procedure has been little studied (and as one might expect, therefore quickly dismissed), the method for preparing the test solution and its administration is included.

A 50 cc. volumetric flask with ground glass stopper is autoclaved at 15 pounds pressure for 15 minutes. The flask is removed, stoppered immediately, and then set aside. Thirty-five cc. of freshly distilled water is heated to boiling in a separate container and allowed to cool to 95° C. A 24 mg. sample of 2, 6-dichlorobenzenoneindophenol (certified reagent of Fischer Scientific Company #5-286) is weighed out on an analytic balance. This sample is added to the 35 cc. of water which is then allowed to cool. Another beaker, containing enough water to dilute the dye solution to 50 cc. is boiled and also allowed to cool. The solution is then transferred to a 50 cc. volumetric flask with rinsings and adjusted to the 50 cc. mark. This then constitutes the intradermal test solution.

The forearm is cleansed with 70 percent alcohol. A 4 mm. area is then marked with a red pen. With a sterile 2 cc. tuberculin syringe and 1/2 inch 25 gauge needle, 0.05 cc. of the dye solution is injected intradermally. This amount of dye is introduced between the marked areas on the forearm producing a wheal 4 mm. in diameter. A stopwatch is immediately set. The decolorization of the wheal is checked periodically to determine the time required for complete decolorization of the reagent.

The number of minutes necessary for total decolorization is referred to as the intradermal ascorbic acid test. The shorter the time required for decolorization, the higher the vitamin C state. Conversely, the longer the time for decolorization, the poorer the vitamin C concentration in the skin.

For more particulars regarding this interesting and not too well known measuring tool, the reader is referred to the Appendix. One can find other publications dealing with this relatively unknown tissue ascorbic acid procedure. A comparison of the skin test and other measures of vitamin C nutriture is also provided.

9.   What is the Lingual Vitamin C Test?

There is general agreement that classical scurvy is rare. However, many authorities insist that marginal (meaning subclinical) deficiency states exist in epidemic proportions. We have reason to agree as evidenced by the material presented in Section A. The Epidemiology of Vitamin C.

Unfortunately, these subtle problems cannot readily be detected by clinical examination. Additionally, the present blood and urine tests for vitamin C status are cumbersome, expensive, difficult to obtain and their interpretation not easy. Thus, simple tools to detect the marginally deficient patient have been needed for a long time. We have looked into the problem of a skin test and this has been reported elsewhere (Question 8, pages 19 and 20).

We have for a long time been concerned with the measurement of ascorbic acid using conventional techniques but always looking for a relatively simple, inexpensive and quick test. This was provided to us in the early 1960s by Giza and his group in Poland and we have been studying quite extensively this procedure with modifications for many years. Our interests and publications in this area are abundantly clear by examining the Appendix.

The technique is very simple. The patient should be seated in an area where the tongue may be directly illuminated. After rinsing the mouth thoroughly with tap water, the protruded tongue should be grasped and held with a gauze pad. With the subject's mouth opened wide, the dorsum of the tongue in the vicinity of the junction of the anterior and middle thirds may be observed. This area is dried with a gauze pad being careful to stroke the papillae so that they stand erect. A papillated area to the left or right of the midline is chosen and one drop of a 1/340 N 2, 6-dicholoroindophenol sodium salt solution is deposited. The correct drop is assured by holding the syringe at approximately a 45° angle. Just as the drop lands upon the tongue, timing is initiated with a stopwatch and timing is continued until the blue color has disappeared. This time period is recorded in seconds.

The Lingual Ascorbic Acid Test time (usually abbreviated LAAT) of approximately 20 seconds or less indicates that the tissue is well supplied with ascorbic acid; 20 to 25 seconds reflects a marginal or suboptimal vitamin C tissue level; and greater than 25 seconds indicates a definite vitamin C deficit.

This story is described in a number of the articles listed in the Appendix. However, one may obtain full particulars about the technique by examining "The Lingual Ascorbic Acid Test" which appeared in Quintessence International (9: #12: 81-85, December 1978).

10. How Does Plasma Ascorbic Acid Correlate With the Lingual Vitamin C Test?

As we have indicated elsewhere, the plasma ascorbic acid concentration is the most popular biochemical measure of ascorbic acid state. We have also indicated our interest in a new and exciting tongue test. The obvious question has to be "how does the plasma ascorbic acid level compare to the lingual vitamin C concentration?".

We have studied this problem a number of years ago in 1194 subjects. The lingual vitamin C test was performed as described elsewhere and the plasma ascorbic acid level was measured by the Mindlin-Butler technique (page 18). The combination of tests was done under fasting conditions in 430 individuals. It was performed under postprandial circumstances in 764 persons.

Table 10.1

correlation of lingual vitamin C test and plasma ascorbic acid concentration

conditions	sample pairs	r	p
fasting	430	-0.3415	<0.01
two-hour postprandial	764	-0.1514	<0.01

Table 10.1 summarizes the correlation coefficients as determined from the lingual vitamin C test scores and the plasma ascorbic acid concentrations. It will be noted that, under both fasting and two-hour postprandial conditions, there is a negative correlation. In other words, the higher the plasma ascorbic acid concentration, the shorter the lingual time. Additionally, Table 10.1 underlines the fact that under fasting and two-hour postprandial circumstances the correlation coefficients are statistically significant at the 1% confidence level. Finally, it will be noted that the correlation coefficient is over twice as great in the fasting studies versus the nonfasting series (-0.3415 versus -0.1514). The differences become more sharply

defined when one compares the fasting and postprandial relationship as spelled out in Tables 10.2 and 10.3. First, under fasting conditions, the various plasma vitamin C groups means are more clearly delineated in the fasting state. Secondly, the standard deviations are smaller under fasting conditions.

Table 10.2

variability in fasting plasma ascorbic acid levels and lingual
vitamin C test scores

lingual time groups (seconds)	sample size	plasma ascorbic acid (mg per cent)	
		mean	standard deviation
0-19	156	0.93	0.30
20-39	208	0.63	0.31
40+	66	0.61	0.30
total	430		

Table 10.3

variability in two-hour postprandial plasma ascorbic acid levels
and lingual vitamin C test scores

lingual time groups (seconds)	sample size	plasma ascorbic acid (mg per cent)	
		mean	standard deviation
0-19	204	0.68	0.34
20-39	467	0.59	0.33
40+	93	0.53	0.35
total	764		

It is abundantly clear, within the limits of this study already reported (A Lingual Vitamin C Test: III. Relationship to Plasma Ascorbic Acid Level. International Journal for Vitamin Research 38: #1, 120-122, 1968), that there is a significant inverse relationship between the lingual test time scores and plasma ascorbic acid levels (Figure 10.1). However, the correlation is by no means perfect. This is very likely due to three reasons. Firstly, there is an experimental error in the performance of the lingual vitamin C test. Secondly, there is also a laboratory error in the measurement of the plasma ascorbic acid level.

Figure 10.1

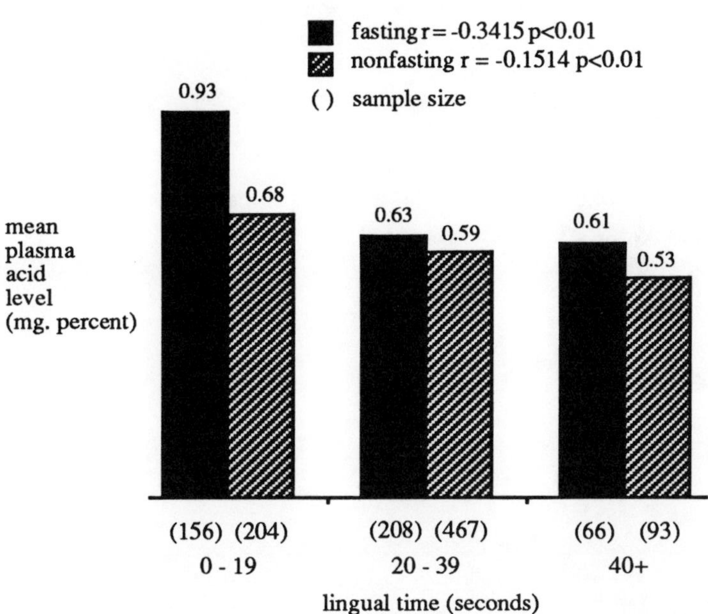

Finally, there is reason to believe that the plasma ascorbic acid level is more a function of dietary intake than tissue saturation. In contrast, the evidence suggests the lingual test time may likely be more reflective of tissue state.

11. How Significant is the Relationship Between Dietary Vitamin C Consumption and Vitamin C Tissue State as Judged by Measurement in the Tongue?

Because of the relative nonavailability of good and quick vitamin C measures and because of our interest in the lingual vitamin C test as an index of tissue vitamin C state, we have naturally been very concerned with determining the validity and reliability of measuring vitamin C in the tongue tissue.

Accordingly, in this particular study, the intent was to examine the sensitivity of the lingual vitamin C test following ascorbic acid versus placebo supplementation. We did just that in an experiment which was subsequently published as "A Lingual Vitamin C Test: VI. Effect of Three Week Vitamin C Versus Placebo Supplementation" in the International Journal for Vitamin Research (38: #2, 257-259, 1968).

Table 11.1

change in lingual test time scores
with placebo versus vitamin C supplementation

	placebo group number and percentage of subjects	vitamin C group number and percentage of subjects
increase	14 (56%)	0 (0%)
no change	3 (12%)	1 (4%)
decrease	8 (32%)	24 (96%)
total	25 (100%)	25 (100%)

Fifty presumably healthy subjects were divided into two groups of 25 each. One subset received thrice daily with meals one capsule containing 100 mg. of milk sugar. In contrast, the other 25 subjects were provided three times daily at meal time with one capsule containing

100 mg. of a synthetic vitamin C preparation. The capsules in both of the subsets were indistinguishable.

The lingual vitamin C test was performed under fasting conditions at the beginning and at the end, meaning following three weeks of supplementation. The means and standard deviations for the lingual times before and after placebo supplementation were strikingly similar (25.9 versus 26.8 seconds). This was clearly not statistically significant. In contrast, the lingual times before and after vitamin C supplementation proved to be 25.8 and 15.7 seconds respectively. This reduction in the lingual time (suggesting improvement in vitamin C state) of an order of 10 seconds and approximately 39% proved to be highly statistically significant.

Viewed another way, namely in terms of number of subjects increasing, decreasing, and showing no change in tissue status, it is clear from the accompanying illustration (Table 10.1) that 96 percent of the subjects improved in tissue ascorbic acid state with vitamin C in contrast to 32 percent who improved with the placebo supplement.

This simple experiment suggests that significant changes in vitamin C state at least as judged in the tongue may be obtained with relatively small amounts of vitamin C and in surprisingly short periods of time.

12. How do the Skin and Tongue Vitamin C Diagnostic Tests Compare?

Clearly, the two tests which have least been utilized for vitamin C measurement have been the intradermal and the tongue procedures. Incidentally, these are the two techniques which we have spent considerable time and energy studying over a number of years. Hence, the obvious question which must be answered is how do the results stemming from these two procedures compare. We utilized 616 subjects for this procedure which led to a publication entitled "A Lingual Vitamin C Test: IV. Relationship to Intradermal Time" which appeared in the International Journal for Vitamin Research (38: #1, 123-126, 1968).

Table 12.1 summarizes the correlation coefficients as determined from the lingual vitamin C test scores and the intradermal test values. It will be noted that, for the entire sample, there is a positive and significant correlation ($r=+0.1865$, $p<0.01$). It will also be observed that, viewed in terms of food intake, only the fasting relationship is statistically significant ($r=+0.4496$, $p<0.01$).

Table 12.1

correlation of intradermal and lingual test time scores

group	sample pairs	r	p
entire sample	616	+0.1865	<0.01*
fasting	299	+0.4496	<0.01*
nonfasting	317	+0.0309	>0.05

The significance of the differences under fasting and nonfasting conditions are heightened by a study of Tables 12.2, 12.3, 12.4. The mean values are more sharply defined in the fasting state. Also, the spread (standard deviation) is approximately one-half as great under fasting conditions.

For example, in the 115 subjects with the best lingual

time (0 to 19 seconds), the standard deviation is 5.7 minutes for the skin time (Table 12.3). In contrast, the

Table 12.2

relationship of intradermal and lingual test time scores (entire sample)

lingual time groups (seconds)	sample size	intradermal time (minutes)	
		mean	standard deviation
0-19	211	27.4	10.0
20-39	325	31.7	10.2
40+	80	32.0	9.5
total	616		

Table 12.3

relationship of intradermal and lingual test time scores (fasting group)

lingual time groups (seconds)	sample size	intradermal time (minutes)	
		mean	standard deviation
0-19	115	22.0	5.7
20-39	139	27.7	6.4
40+	45	29.8	9.2
total	299		

Table 12.4

relationship of intradermal and lingual test time scores (nonfasting group)

lingual time groups (seconds)	sample size	intradermal time (minutes)	
		mean	standard deviation
0-19	98	33.6	10.2
20-39	139	34.7	11.5
40+	34	34.9	9.4
total	317		

standard deviation for those with the same lingual time under nonfasting conditions is 10.2 for the skin test (Table 12.4)

Finally, it is well to summarize the relationships between the lingual test times, the intradermal scores, and plasma ascorbic acid concentration (Table 12.5). It is

Table 12.5

relationships of lingual vitamin C test, intradermal test and plasma ascorbic acid

comparison	conditions	sample size	r	p
lingual vitamin C test versus intradermal time	fasting	299	+0.4496	<0.01*
lingual vitamin C test versus plasma ascorbic acid	fasting	430	-0.3415	<0.01*
lingual vitamin C test versus plasma ascorbic acid	nonfasting	264	-0.1514	<0.01*
lingual vitamin C test versus intradermal time	nonfasting	317	+0.0309	>0.05

* statistically significant

evident that the highest correlation (r=+0.4496, p<0.01) prevails between the fasting lingual and intradermal times. In other words, the longer the lingual time; the longer the intradermal time. The next most significant (p<0.01) correlation (r=-0.3415) exists between the fasting lingual time and fasting plasma ascorbic acid. Thus, the longer the lingual time; the lower the plasma ascorbic acid concentration. It is noteworthy that the two relationships with the highest correlation are under fasting conditions. Finally, mention should be made that the only correlation which is not significant (p>0.05) is found between the nonfasting intradermal and lingual times.

Overall, and within the limits of this simple study there do indeed appear to be relationships of a significant nature between the various vitamin C modality testing procedures.

13. How Sensitive is Vitamin C Nutriture to Dietary Intake?

An inspection of the Appendix will quickly confirm our long concern with three reflections of vitamin C state, namely (1) the traditional plasma ascorbic acid level testing technique, (2) the less known and less understood intradermal decolorization time and (3) lingual vitamin C test technique.

We have been very curious for some time to ascertain which of these procedures is reflective and to what degree of dietary intake as measured by daily orange consumption, daily orange juice intake, and vitamin C supplementation.

Herein are the answers derived from a story of 262 subjects. All of the participants were examined in terms

Table 13.1

relationship of fasting vitamin C state and vitamin consumption			
	negative	positive	p
daily orange juice consumption			
plasma ascorbic acid	0.6	0.8	<0.001*
intradermal time	29.3	26.0	>0.050
lingual time	29.3	24.1	<0.010*
daily orange consumption			
plasma ascorbic acid	0.7	0.7	>0.500
intradermal time	27.8	26.2	>0.400
lingual time	25.7	27.5	>0.400
daily vitamin supplement			
plasma ascorbic acid	0.7	0.9	<0.001*
intradermal time	28.5	23.9	<0.025*
lingual time	28.4	19.7	<0.001*

* statistically significant

of vitamin C state as measured by plasma ascorbic acid level, intradermal decolorization test time, and lingual test scores in the fasting state in 102 (Table 13.1) of the group and under nonfasting, that is postprandial conditions, in 160 persons (Table 13.2).

The daily intake of citrus juices, oranges, and vitamin C supplementation were compared with plasma ascorbic acid levels, intradermal times, and lingual vitamin C test scores for the entire sample of 262 subjects.

Table 13.1 is a summary of our observations reported in "A Lingual Vitamin C Test: V. A Study in Dietary Relationships" which was released in the International Journal for Vitamin Research (38: #2, 254-256, 1968).

Table 13.2

relationship of nonfasting vitamin C state and vitamin consumption

	negative	positive	p
daily orange juice consumption			
plasma ascorbic acid	0.3	0.6	<0.001*
intradermal time	39.1	32.6	<0.001*
lingual time	27.9	25.4	>0.100
daily orange consumption			
plasma ascorbic acid	0.5	0.6	<0.025*
intradermal time	35.9	30.2	<0.025*
lingual time	26.4	26.2	>0.500
daily vitamin supplement			
plasma ascorbic acid	0.4	0.7	<0.001*
intradermal time	35.8	30.7	<0.025*
lingual time	26.3	27.3	>0.500

* statistically significant

For clarification, "negative" indicates that the particular dietary element was not available on a daily basis. For example, negative orange juice consumption simply means that individuals did not take orange juice on a daily basis. In contrast, "positive" indicates that individuals did indeed consume orange juice on a daily basis.

In summary, Table 13.1 shows that, in those consuming and not consuming orange juice daily, the plasma ascorbic acid levels and the lingual times are statistically significantly different. Specifically, in those consuming orange juice on a daily basis, the plasma level is statistically higher (0.6 versus 0.8 mg. percent). With regard to daily orange consumption, it will be noted from the illustration that there is no difference in the plasma levels, the intradermal times or the lingual times. Finally, it is also evident that in the subjects consuming a daily vitamin supplement there is a statistically significant difference in plasma ascorbic acid levels, intradermal times and lingual scores versus those not consuming a vitamin supplement.

Table 13.2 summarizes similar relationships of the various vitamin C parameters under nonfasting conditions. In all instances, the lingual vitamin C test times are not statistically significant.

Hence, overall, there are indeed interesting and significant reflections of dietary consumption as judged by these three different vitamin C measuring sticks. Additionally, there are minor differences in whether the measurements are derived under fasting or nonfasting conditions.

Summarizing the findings in another way, the evidence suggests that, in general, there is a correlation between vitamin C state and daily vitamin C consumption in the 262 presumably healthy subjects reported in this experiment. The evidence suggests that, in general, there is a correlation between vitamin C state and daily vitamin C intake. This is particularly true under fasting conditions and more especially so when plasma ascorbic acid is utilized as the vitamin C measure. One parenthetic note. This is additional support for the argument that plasma ascorbic acid concentration is more a measure of dietary than tissue state.

<u>PART</u>

<u>THREE</u>

<u>VITAMIN</u>

<u>C</u>

<u>IN</u>

<u>GENERAL</u>

<u>HEALTH</u>

<u>AND</u>

<u>DISEASE</u>

Many lives would be saved if the medicine chest contained ascorbic acid in place of aspirin and other cold medicines.

Dr. Linus Pauling
Vitamin C and the
Common Cold 1970

14. Are There Overall Known Correlations Between Vitamin C and General Health?

There are many publications dealing with **specific** relationships between vitamin C and health and sickness. As far as we can determine, there was not then (nor is there now) any overall portrayal of the possible connection of vitamin C and the sickness/wellness modality.

We presented our thoughts on this matter at the Eighth Biomedical Engineering Symposium in San Diego in 1974 and our presentation was subsequently published in the Proceedings of the San Diego Biomedical Symposium in Volume 13 in a presentation entitled "The Name of the Game is the Name" (Proceedings San Diego Biomedical Symposium 1974. 13: 31-39, 6/8 February 1974).

Table 14.1

distribution of daily vitamin C consumption (seven-day survey)

vitamin C group	number of subjects	percentage of subjects
0- 44	74	6.8
45- 90	220	20.3
91-180	537	49.4
181-269	189	17.4
270+	66	6.1
total	1086	100.0
mean		140.3
S.D.		80.5
minimum		4
maximum		666
range		662

The data for this study stems from a survey of the health of health professionals which we had been conducting for a number of years. More precisely, we had at that time been engaged in a multiphasic testing program of 1086 doctors and their spouses over an eight-year period.

Table 14.1 summarizes the distribution of vitamin C on a daily basis as judged from a seven-day dietary survey. It is abundantly evident that the mean and standard deviation is 140.3 ± 80.5 mgs. with a minimum of 4 and a maximum of 666 and with a range of 662.

It is safe to conclude that no clinical scurvy was identified in this group. In other words, there is no evidence to suggest that pathosis describing the classical case could be identified in any of these doctors or their spouses. However, clearly, with daily vitamin C intakes as low as 4 mg., there is the suggestion of possible subclinical or marginal vitamin C deficiency.

Figure 14.1

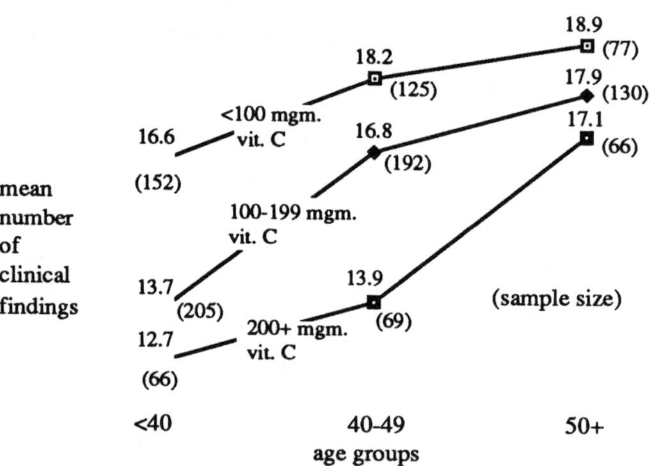

Figure 14.1 depicts the relationship between clinical symptoms and signs pictured on the ordinate in terms of age as described on the abscissa and in the light of daily vitamin C intake. It is clear that the group characterized by the lowest ascorbic acid consumption (less than 100 mg. per day) shows, in all age groups, the greatest number of clinical symptoms and signs, specifically 16.6, 18.2,

and 18.9 respectively. Conversely, the group representing the highest vitamin C intake (200+ mgs. daily) is associated with the least clinical pathosis at all temporal points (12.7, 13.9, and 17.1).

Finally, the group occupying an intermediate position in terms of daily vitamin C intake (100 to 199 mg.), occupies an intermediate place in terms of clinical symptoms and signs (13.7, 16.8, and 17.9).

The point of this story, as underlined by this particular exercise, is that the present health and disease patterns become more meaningful when one discards the traditional disease classification (in this case, the syndrome of scurvy) for the earliest evidence of the syndrome of sickness (clinical symptoms and signs). Additionally, this becomes more meaningful when one grants that small differences in vitamin C intake may be viewed as one mistake in lifestyle.

Surprisingly, this is one of a few published reports in the literature dealing with the overall problem of health and sickness versus ascorbic acid. Clearly, much is still to be done. However, within the limits of this experiment and recognizing the restraints of correlations, it seems that vitamin C serves a ubiquitous role in health and sickness.

Perhaps the most dramatic way of answering this question has already been done in a paper entitled "The Name of the Game is the Name: A Second and Harder Look" which appeared in the Journal of Holistic Medicine (6: 73-79, 1981). The greatest amount of vitamin C (200+ mg. per day) clinically parallels the 40-year-old with the least amount of vitamin C intake. This is underlined in Figure 14.1 showing that those 50+ year-old subjects taking 200+ mg. of vitamin C per day report 17.1 complaints which is less than the 18.2 complaints in those 40 to 49-year-old subjects consuming less than 100 mg. of vitamin C per day. This is simply another way of explaining the oft-heard question as to why some people are 40 going on 60 and others are 60 going on 40!

15. What about Vitamin C Consumption and Respiratory Findings?

Since 1970, a considerable body of fact, admittedly still in debate, has been published regarding the possible relationship between ascorbic acid and the common cold.

We have not looked at this particular problem for a number of reasons including the fact that it is extremely difficult to identify the endpoints of a common cold. For example, when is the common cold no longer a common cold but influenza, or bronchitis, or pneumonitis? For

Figure 15.1

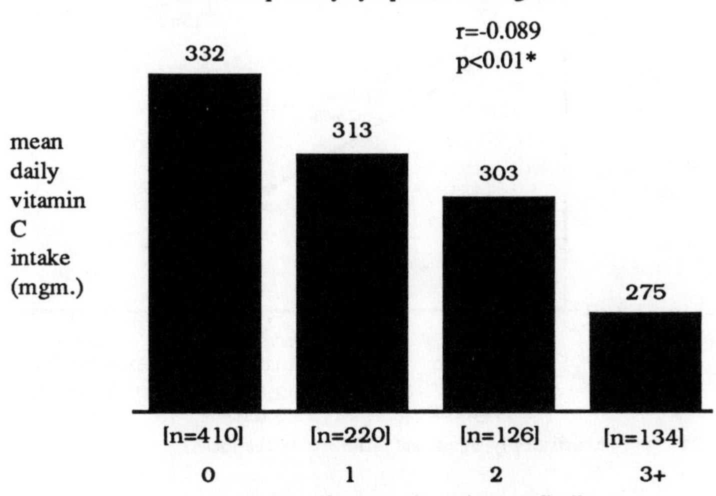

these and other reasons, we have been more interested in analyzing the possible relationship between daily vitamin C consumption and overall respiratory findings which, one can safely say, are surely more measurable. For example, it is relatively easy to identify whether an individual spits up blood or has a sharp pain in the chest with coughing, etc.

Eight hundred and ninety dental practitioners and their spouses were studied on one occasion in terms of

Figure 15.2

changes in reported respiratory symptoms and signs at three annual examination periods in those who at the third examination are consuming <400 versus 400+ mg vitamin C per day

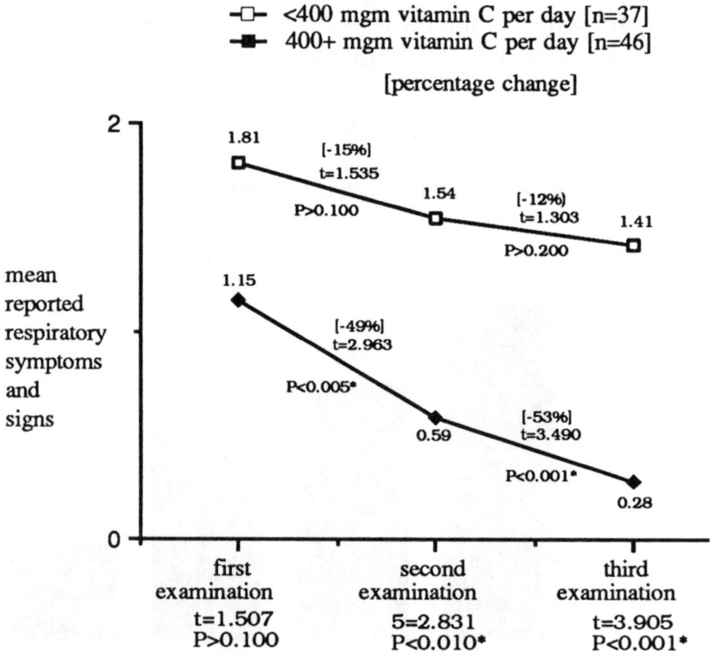

* statistically significant difference of the means

reported daily vitamin C consumption versus reported respiratory symptoms and signs. From this group, 83 subjects were subsequently reexamined one and two years later following group nutritional seminars.

Figure 15.1 pictures the relationship between the frequency of reported respiratory symptoms and signs (on the abscissa) versus the daily vitamin C intake (on the ordinate). The chart shows clearly that those 410 subjects with no respiratory complaints seem to be the very ones with the mean highest daily vitamin C intake (332 mg.). In contrast, the 134 subjects with the 3+ respiratory findings enjoy the lowest mean ascorbic acid consumption (275 mg.). The intermediate groups in terms of respiratory complaints are paralleled by intermediate scores of daily vitamin C consumption.

On a mean basis, it will be noted that there is a progressive decline in respiratory findings in parallel with an increase in daily vitamin C consumption. It is also clear that there is a low but statistically significant correlation coefficient (r=-0.089, p<0.01) meaning that the higher the daily vitamin C consumption, the fewer the respiratory findings.

Figure 15.2 summarizes the mean reported symptoms and signs (on the ordinate) at the first, second, and third examinations (on the abscissa). Additionally, the sample has been divided into those who, at the third examination, were consuming <400 mgs. of vitamin C per day (37 subjects pictured by the open rectangles) versus those who were consuming 400+ mgs. vitamin C on a daily basis (46 subjects shown by the dark squares).

Five points warrant special mention. First, on a mean basis, there is a reduction in respiratory complaints in both subgroups. Second, also on a mean basis, the decline in respiratory findings is greater in those who at the third examination, are consuming the greater amounts (400+ mgs.) of vitamin C. Third, there appears to be no statistically significant difference (t=1.507, p>0.100) at the start of the study (not shown in the illustration). Fourthly, while the groups are not substantially different at the beginning, they do indeed become progressively more different at the second and at the third examinations.

Finally, there are no statistically significant differences in the lower (<400 mg.) vitamin C intake group between the first and second visits as shown by t=1.535, p>0.100 and a t=1.303, p>0.200. In sharp contrast, there are very clearcut decrements in the group characterized by the greater daily vitamin C consumption at the second and third visit. This is underlined by the t=2.963, p<0.005 and t=3.490, p<0.001.

Thus, in answer to this final question, the most notable reduction in respiratory symptoms and signs seems to have occurred in the group characterized by the greater daily ascorbic acid consumption. Parenthetic mention should be made that the greater daily vitamin C intake is considerably greater than the recommended dietary allowances.

This report entitled "Vitamin C Consumption and Reported Respiratory Findings" was published in the International Journal for Vitamin and Nutrition Research (43: #1, 42-55, 1973) during the heat of the controversy regarding the relationship of vitamin C to the common cold. While the problems have many characteristics which make them very different, there are many commonalities. In a sense, they both support the notion that there might well be a relationship between ascorbic acid consumption and respiratory disease in general and, therefore, vitamin C and the common cold in particular.

16. Can One Identify Any Possible Connection Between Vitamin C and Cardiovascular Symptomatology?

One thousand and seventy-four dental practitioners and their spouses were initially evaluated between 1965 and 1972 in terms of their dietary patterns and reported clinical state. Included in this longstanding health evaluation was a clinical score for cardiovascular symptoms and signs derived from the Cornell Medical Index Health Questionnaire. The daily vitamin C consumption was ascertained from a food frequency questionnaire.

It became abundantly clear early in the study that many of the participants were consuming large amounts of refined carbohydrate foodstuffs, suboptimal amounts of protein, and relatively small quantities of vitamins and minerals. The therapeutic regimen consisted of a series of brief nutritional seminars demonstrating to the group their dietary deficits and avenues for dietary improvement.

With regard to this particular part of the survey, an attempt was made to answer five questions. First, what is the frequency of reported cardiovascular findings in such a presumably healthy population? In answer to this question, cardiovascular symptomatology was found to range from 0 to 9 complaints with a mean of 1.21.

Secondly, what is the daily vitamin C consumption in this same type of group? According to the Recommended Dietary Allowances, these subjects were consuming approximately four to five times more vitamin C than officially recommended which, at that time, was 60 mg. for the male and 55 mg. for the female per day. Specifically, at the initial evaluation, the values were 294 ± 180 mg. of vitamin C per day extending from a minimum of 15 to a maximum of 881 mg.

Thirdly, could one identify any relationship between the frequency of reported cardiovascular symptoms and signs and daily ascorbic acid consumption? In answer to this third question, it was clear that there is a low but statistically significant negative correlation meaning that

48

the higher the daily vitamin C consumption, the fewer the cardiovascular findings. Figure 16.1 pictorially portrays the relationship. For example, the 468 subjects with no cardiovascular complaints consumed, on the average, 338 mgs. of vitamin C per day. In contrast, the 133 participants with 3+ cardiovascular symptoms and signs consumed 308 mgs. of vitamin C per day. The intermediate groups

Figure 16.1

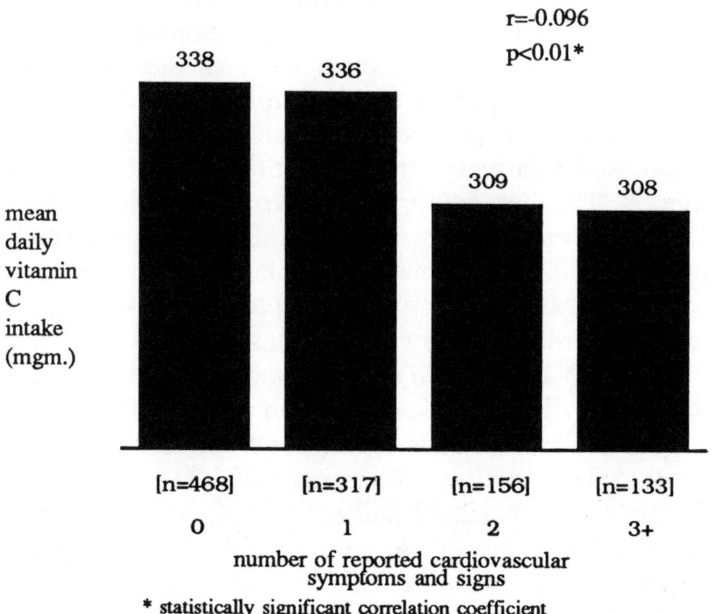

in terms of cardiovascular symptomatology were represented by intermediate amounts of daily vitamin C consumption. Hence, in answer to this third question, it seems clear that there is a low but statistically significant negative correlation (r=-0.096, p<0.01).

Fourthly, an attempt was made to answer the question as to what changes if any in the frequency of reported cardiovascular symptoms and signs occur following a one-year experimental period during which group nutritional improvement instructions were conducted? Parenthetic mention should be made that well over three-fourths, actually 77.8 percent of the group increased daily ascorbic acid intake between the first and second annual

Figure 16.2

relationship of change in daily vitamin C intake food frequency questionnaire to change in reported cardiovascular findings (CMI)

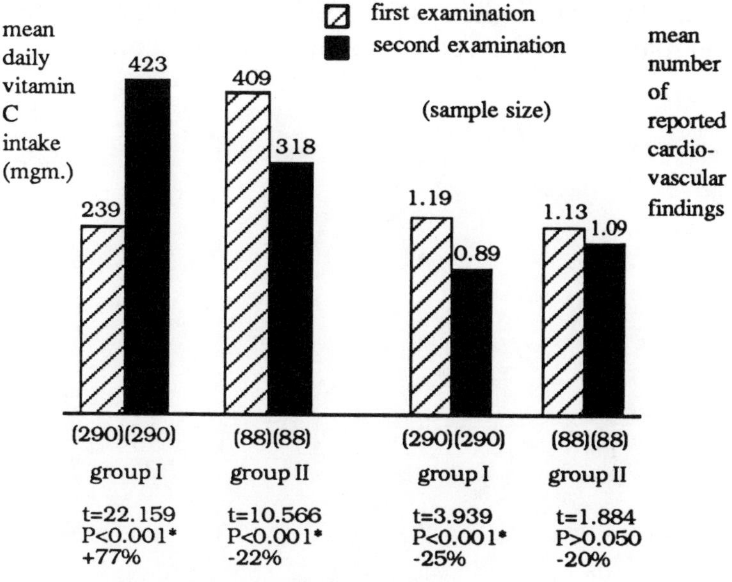

sessions. In parallel, the mean cardiovascular score was reduced from 1.19 to 0.89 cardiovascular symptoms and signs per subject (Figure 16.2).

Viewed another way, the 290 subjects who chose to increase their daily vitamin C intake actually increased it from 239 to 423 mg. The cardiovascular score decreased, as has already been mentioned, from 1.19 to 0.89. This also proved to be highly statistically significant (t=3.939, p<0.001). In contrast, a second group of 88 individuals chose not to increase their vitamin C consumption. Actually, the daily intake decreased from 409 to 318 mg. per day. Interestingly in this group, there was no statistically significant change in the reported cardiovascular picture.

This problem was studied in great detail and more particulars may be obtained from the original paper entitled "Daily Vitamin C Consumption and Reported Cardiovascular Findings" which was released in the Journal of the International Academy of Preventive Medicine (1: #1, 31-44, Spring 1974).

While most of the information in that report suggests an interesting correlation, it should be pointed out that some of the data indicates the possibility that this correlation may indeed be of a cause-and-effect nature.

17. Vitamin C Consumption and Fatigability?

It has long been known, actually since about 1750, that sailors on long voyages frequently became fatigued and eventually died. Additionally, in the famous Crandon classic study of 1940, one of the first evidences of experimental human scurvy proved to be a progressive feeling of fatigue which developed in approximately 90 days. Finally, it is a matter of record that one of the most common presenting complaints in the offices of health practitioners has been variously labeled as fatigue, exhaustion, tiredness.

Parenthetic mention should be made that, in a recent study by the Department of Health and Human Services, it was discovered that fatigability is one of America's most common presenting complaints.

In view of these known earlier facts, ascorbic acid consumption was determined in 411 dentists and their spouses from a simple food frequency questionnaire. Additionally, the number of fatigue symptoms listed in the answers to seven questions comprising Section I of the Cornell Medical Index Health Questionnaire were utilized. The relationship between these two variables was determined by calculating the fatigability score for different levels of daily vitamin C consumption. This material was put together and released as "Daily Vitamin C Consumption and Fatigability" and subsequently published in the Journal of the American Geriatrics Society (24: #3, 136-137, 1976).

It was discovered that the 81 subjects who consumed less than 100 mg. of vitamin C per day recorded a fatigability score of 0.81. Conversely, the 330 subjects consuming more than 400 mg. of vitamin C on a daily basis reported a fatigability score of 0.41. Parenthetically, this two-fold difference proved to be statistically significant suggesting that those persons consuming greater amounts of vitamin C tend to display less fatigability.

18.   Is There any Possible Connection Between Vitamin C and the Skin?

It is noteworthy that the number of persons with one or more skin conditions comes to a staggering 25,000,000 in the civilian noninstitutionalized population of the United States according to the best estimates we have from the United States Department of Health and Human Services.   Since this figure has been relatively constant

Figure 18.1

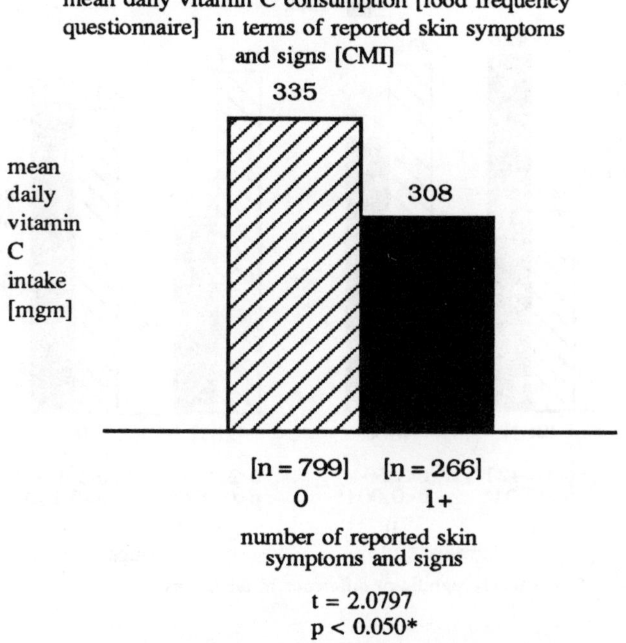

during the recent years, it would suggest that the diverse traditional therapies have not served as the solution. It is quite probable that factors relating to the cause, cure, and prevention of skin disorders have been overlooked or carelessly discarded or both.

In an attempt to identify heretofore unrecognized variables in the genesis of skin disorders, dietary and medical histories of 1065 doctors and their spouses were analyzed including daily vitamin C consumption. Some of this material was put together and eventually published as "Relationship of Vitamin C and Skin Symptoms and Signs" in the Journal of the Canadian Chiropractic Association (22: #3, 97-98, October 1978).

Figure 18.2

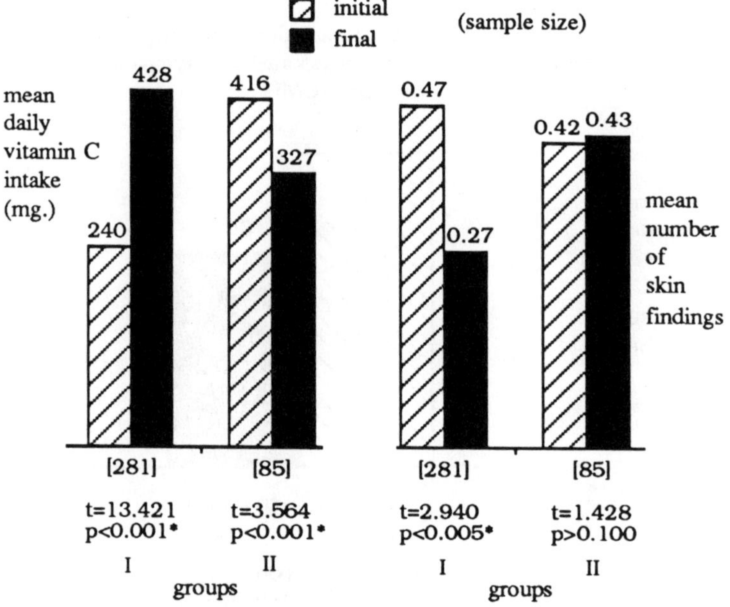

Figure 18.1 demonstrates that the consumption of ascorbic acid was found to be significantly related to the number of reported skin symptoms and signs. Specifically, the mean daily vitamin C intake was 335 mg. per day in the 799 subjects with no reported skin symptoms and signs. This is emphasized by the striped column. In contrast, the mean daily vitamin C intake was 308 mg. in

the 266 individuals with one or more reported skin symptoms and signs (black column). This difference, as shown in Figure 18.1, is highly significant (t=2.0797, p<0.050). However, it should be quickly emphasized that the mere fact that this relationship prevails does not necessarily prove a cause-and-effect pattern.

Accordingly, the mean number of skin findings were analyzed at the beginning and at the end of a one-year period in two groups differing in their change in daily vitamin C consumption (Figure 18.2). Specifically, one group consisted of 281 subjects who increased their daily vitamin C intake, on the average, from 240 to 428 mg. per day. In this group, the mean number of skin findings decreased approximately 50 percent. In contrast, in 85 subjects who did not increase and, in fact, slightly decreased their daily vitamin C intake from 416 to 327 mg. per day, there was no statistically significant change in the mean number of skin findings.

Hence, this report proposes a significant positive association of vitamin C and skin disorders. What this report suggests actually is that there is some evidence to indicate that those subjects who increased their daily vitamin C intake significantly reduced the number of skin findings. Conversely, those persons who did not increase their daily vitamin C consumption showed no significant change in the mean number of integumentary symptoms and signs.

19. Are There Known Relationships Between Vitamin C and the Electrocardiogram?

There is now complete agreement that heart disease is one of the major killing and crippling syndromes of the twentieth century. There is also no argument but that heart disease is polygenic and that diet plays a role. However, within this area, major consideration has been given to fats and increasing importance is being assigned to refined carbohydrate foods. Finally, the original stories of scurvy described in the 1750s by Surgeon Captain James Lind (generally not cited) noted the fact that scorbutic subjects frequently succumbed with congestive heart failure. Notwithstanding this historic and admittedly anecdotal information, we have been unable to identify experiments relating any of the numerous electrocardiographic parameters to vitamin C state. It was that that led us to look at the problem which we subsequently reported as "Electrocardiography and Vitamin C: P-Wave Height (Lead I)" in the Journal of the International Academy of Preventive Medicine (6: #2, 11-20, 1981).

In 1965, a multiple health testing program for members of the health professions was inaugurated under the auspices of the Southern Academy of Clinical Nutrition. In 1969, the project was extended to include a group designated as the Southern California Academy of Nutrition Research, and a third group was organized under the aegis of the Ohio Academy of Clinical Nutrition. In 1971, a fourth segment was added under the direction of the Northeast Academy of Clinical Nutrition. Finally, in 1972, a fifth group was started under the guidance of the Northern California Academy of Nutritional Research.

Seven hundred and fourteen dental practitioners and their spouses were evaluated initially between 1965 and 1972 in terms of dietary pattern as well as electrocardiography. The daily vitamin C intake was obtained from a food frequency questionnaire. It became clear that many of the participants were consuming large amounts of refined carbohydrate foodstuffs, suboptimal amounts of protein and relatively small amounts of vitamins and minerals.

The therapeutic regimen consisted of several brief nutritional seminars showing the dietary deficits and measures for dietary improvement.

This experiment was designed to answer three questions. First, what is the relationship between the height of P1 and age? Table 19.1 outlines the relationship of age in the two sexes and the height of the P wave in Lead I. It will be noted that, with advancing age in the male, the means rise from 0.49 to 0.51 to 0.57 mm.; in the female, the scores with advancing age are 0.48, 0.51 and 0.52 mm. Hence, in answer to this first question, there appears to be a rise in the height of P1 with advancing age in both sexes and presumably a greater increase in the male group.

The second question raises the point "are there parallelisms between vitamin C intake and the height of P1?" The 75 subjects consuming less than 100 mg. per day of vitamin C were found to have a P1 height of 0.607 ± 0.266 mm (Table 19.2). In contrast, the 331 subjects consuming greater than 400 mg. per day of vitamin C displayed a P1 height of 0.440 ± 0.221. This 27.5 percentage change is highly significant as shown by $t=5.063$ and a $p<0.001$.

Table 19.1

relationship of P-wave height (Lead I) and age in a presumably healthy male and female sample

age groups	male			female		
	n	mean age	mean height P_1	n	mean age	mean height P_1
40	156	34.0	0.49	160	31.8	0.48
40-49	153	44.0	0.51	94	43.7	0.51
50+	98	56.4	0.57	53	56.9	0.52

Hence, in response to the second question, there seems no doubt but that there are indeed statistically significant relationships between the height of P1 and daily vitamin C consumption. Specifically, the height of P1 is less in those consuming the greater amount of vitamin C.

Table 19.2

relationship of daily vitamin C intake and electrocardiography

	n	low vitamin C <100 mg./day	n	high vitamin C >400 mg./day	percent-age change	t	p
height P1	75	0.607	331	0.440	27.5	5.063	<0.001*

And finally, are there changes in the height of P1 associated with changes in vitamin C intake? An attempt was made to study the changes in the height of P1 in terms of the changes in daily vitamin C intake (Table 19.3). For example, 268 subjects were randomly chosen who increased their vitamin C consumption during a one-year period. The initial range consisted of 16 to 723 mg. per day with a mean and a standard deviation of 236.4±134.5. The final values were found to range from 49 to 885 with a mean and a standard deviation of 417.1±181.1. This increase of 43.3 percent is obviously statistically significant (t=21.200, p<0.001) because the group was so chosen. In this sample characterized by an increase in vitamin C, the 268 subjects showed an initial range of P-wave height in Lead I of 0.10 to 1.60 with a mean and standard deviation of 0.53±0.26. The final scores ranged from 0.10 to 1.35 with a mean and standard deviation of 0.46±0.24. This 14.0 percent reduction is statistically highly significant (t=5.73, p<0.001). In contrast, Table 19.3 shows 75 individuals characterized by a decrease in vitamin C. The initial range was between 78 and 727 mg. per day with a mean and standard deviation of 401.3±182.0. The final range was between 42 and 618 with a mean and standard deviation of 317.3±146.6. The percentage reduction of 21.0 is statistically significant (5=9.353, p<0.001). The P-wave height in the 75 subjects ranged initially from 0.15 to 0.90 with a mean and standard deviation of 0.51±0.19. The final range was between 0.10 and 0.90 with a mean and standard deviation of 0.46±0.05. The percentage decline of 9.2 is not statistically significant (t=1.890, p>0.050). Hence, with regard to the third and final question, the subjects characterized by an increase in vitamin C demonstrated a decrease in P-wave height in Lead I; conversely, those subjects with a decrease in vitamin C showed no significant change in P-wave height in Lead I.

Table 19.3

relationship of changes in P-wave height (Lead I) in terms of changes in daily vitamin C intake

group characterized by increase in vitamin C	n	initial examination range	mean	final examination range	mean	percentage change	t	p
vitamin C	268	16-723	236.4	49-885	417.1	+43.3	21.200	<0.001*
P-wave height (Lead I)	268	0.10-1.60	0.53	0.10-1.35	0.46	-14.0	5.173	<0.001*
group characterized by decrease in vitamin C								
vitamin C	75	78-727	401.3	42-618	317.3	-21.0	9.353	<0.001*
P-wave height (Lead I)	75	0.15-0.90	0.51	0.10-0.90	0.46	-9.2	1.890	>0.050

* statistically significant difference of the means

Other electrocardiographic parameters have also been studied; specifically, the length of the P-wave in Lead I has been reported in an article entitled "A Relationship Between Vitamin C Intake and Electrocardiography" which appeared in the Journal of Electrocardiology (12: #4, 441, 1979).

20. Can Contact Lens Intolerance be Altered with Vitamin C Intake?

There is no question but that the contact lens business is a multibillion dollar industry. According to the best available figures, the total number of Americans wearing contact lenses is somewhere between 19.5 and 22 million. The usual figure cited is approximately 20.5 million. The total sales at the manufacturers' level is approximately $480 million which is putatively an increase of about 5% over the previous year. This number translates into about $1.3 billion in sales at the retail level. It is the conventional wisdom in the business that most contact lens patients are those who are constantly being refitted when new materials or new designs are introduced. These figures and others suggest that the **real** success factor is not excellent. It is fair to say that it varies considerably with the eye condition, the age of the patient, and the proper patient selection by the professional. There are no hard data regarding the success factor in contact lens fitting although some authorities seem to agree that the most successful fitting of people with presbyopia with bifocal contact lenses is less than 20%!

Obviously, in some cases, the characteristics of the lens is the prime or most important reason for the failure. It is for this very reason that there is a constant effort to improve the quality of the lens as judged by the hard and soft lens eras, the breathing and non-breathing varieties and now problems with extended wear.

However, in many instances of contact lens failure or intolerance, there do not seem to be any obvious reasons. Phrased another way, the factor which has not been studied in contact lens success versus failure is the ability of the individual to cope with this admittedly foreign agent. And a contact lens is indeed a foreign agent! Defining the ingredients of poor copability or inadequate resistance might well help to answer the question as to why seemingly similar patients supplied with seemingly similar contact lenses prescribed under the supervision of the same eye physician, so often fare so differently.

It was this that led us to look into this matter and to publish a paper entitled "Vitamin C and Contact Lens Intolerance: A Preliminary Report" which was released in the Southern Journal of Optometry (22: #5, 6-8, May 1980).

For this study, thirty-five presumably healthy chiropractic physicians at a scientific meeting, who had been fitted for contact lenses were queried with regard to success or failure in tolerating the lenses. Ten reported success; 25 stated they could not wear them or could only wear them for short periods of time.

The vitamin C state was determined in each subject by the Lingual Ascorbic Acid Test (frequently abbreviated LAAT). The test procedure begins by placing a drop of a blue solution on the dorsum of the tongue. Timing the reaction (preferably by stopwatch) begins immediately after the drop lands on the tissue of the tongue and continues until the blue color has vanished. The recorded number of seconds may be referred to as the Lingual Ascorbic Acid Test (LAAT) time. A LAAT time of 20 seconds or less indicates the tissue is reasonably well supplied with vitamin C; 20 to 25 seconds reflects a marginal or suboptimal tissue ascorbic acid concentration; greater than 25 seconds signifies a definite vitamin C deficit.

More particulars regarding this simple vitamin C test are available in a number of articles listed in the Appendix.

The 10 subjects wearing contact lenses successfully showed a range of scores from 15 to 25 seconds with a mean and standard deviation of 17.1 ± 3.0 seconds. In contrast, the 25 individuals wearing contact lenses unsuccessfully showed a range of 15 to 30 seconds and a mean and standard deviation of 23.0 ± 5.0 seconds. The difference between these two groups proved to be statistically significant.

Hence, the findings in this simple preliminary report suggest a possible relationship between contact lens success and vitamin C measured by the lingual vitamin C tissue test. Clearly, this is a preliminary report designed to encourage others to look into this matter more extensively.

21. Is the Relationship of Chronologic to Bone Age in Any Way Dependent upon Vitamin C?

For a number of years we busied ourselves with a series of experiments designed to analyze the relationship between vitamin C and growth and maturation. The purpose of this particular experiment was to examine the possible relationship of chronologic and bone age in terms of vitamin C state by answering three questions. First, what is the relationship of chronologic and bone age in a routine sample of presumably healthy orthodontic patients? Secondly, what is the vitamin C state of this same population? Finally, is the correlation between the chronologic and bone age in any way a function of vitamin C state?

Bone age (BA) was determined from a hand and wrist radiograph in 152 children awaiting orthodontic treatment. Chronologic age (CA) also was recorded in months. Vitamin C was ascertained in the same group of children by means of plasma ascorbic acid levels and the lingual vitamin C test times.

This material was compiled and presented as "Vitamin C and Chronologic Versus Bone Age" which appeared in the Journal of Oral Medicine (28: #3, 77-80, July/September 1973).

With regard to the first question, the chronologic age (CA) and the bone age (BA) are quite similar in this sample of children. This is confirmed overall by statistically significant positive correlation ($r=+0.878$, $p<0.01$).

While there is an overall statistically significant correlation, there are obviously considerable discrepancies between bone age (BA) and chronologic age (CA). This is clearly shown in the chart (Table 21.1). In only 3.5 percent of the group is the relationship perfect, meaning no difference. For example, in one subject (0.7 percent) the bone age is less than the chronologic age by 41 to 50 months. In 2.1 percent, namely 3 subjects, the bone age is greater than the chronologic age up to 31 to 40 months.

Obviously, shades of grey of discrepancy are also included.

At the time we did the study, the recommendations by the Interdepartmental Committee on Nutrition for National Defense (ICNND), plasma ascorbic acid levels less than 0.1 mg. percent were viewed as frankly deficient and 0.2 mg. percent as low.

Utilizing these criteria, it must be concluded that 17.3 percent of the group display suboptimal vitamin C state. However, other authorities contend that 0.6 mg. percent should be the delineation between satisfactory and unsatisfactory state. On this basis, more than half (53.3 percent) of the group demonstrate suboptimal plasma ascorbic acid levels. This is underscored in the accompanying chart (Table 21.2).

Table 21.1

relationships between chronologic age (CA) and bone age (BA)

	difference in months	subjects	
		number	percentage
BA less than CA	41-50	1	0.7
	31-40	2	1.4
	21-30	11	7.7
	11-20	20	14.1
	1-10	30	21.1
BA equal to CA	0	5	3.5
BA greater than CA	1-10	39	20.4
	11-20	34	24.0
	21-30	7	5.0
	31-40	3	2.1
total		152	100.0*

* approximate

According to the best available evidence, the physiologic range for the lingual vitamin C test is approximately 15 to 25 seconds. On this basis, about 55 percent of the subjects display marginal to poor vitamin C state (Table 21.3). Hence, in answer to the second question, apparently a significant segment of this presumably healthy group show suboptimal vitamin C blood or tissue state by one or the other or both of these biochemical standards.

Finally, it is noteworthy and not shown here, the children with the longer lingual times (40+ seconds), suggesting the poorer vitamin C state demonstrate a lower mean positive correlation between chronologic and bone age (r=+0.806) than for the entire group (r=+0.878). Also,

Table 21.2

plasma ascorbic acid frequency distribution

plasma ascorbic acid groups (mg. per cent)	number and percentage of subjects
0.00-0.19	24 (17.3%)
0.20-0.39	29 (20.9%)
0.40-0.59	21 (15.1%)
0.60-0.79	23 (16.5%)
0.80-0.99	14 (10.1%)
1.00+	14 (10.1%)
total	139 (100.0%)

those with the shorter lingual times (<20 seconds) suggesting a relatively good vitamin C state, have a higher mean positive correlation (r=+0.897) than for the entire group.

Hence the evidence suggests, though it would certainly be helpful to have more information, that there may well be greater harmony between chronologic and bone age in those subjects with the better vitamin C nutriture.

Table 21.3

lingual vitamin C test scores distribution

lingual vitamin C scores (seconds)	number and percentage of subjects
10-14	5 (3.6%)
15-19	34 (24.5%)
20-24	25 (18.0%)
25-29	32 (23.0%)
30-34	15 (10.8%)
35-39	12 (9.8%)
40-44	7 (5.0%)
45-49	2 (1.4%)
50-60	7 (5.0%)
total	139 (100.0%)*

* approximate

22.   Time Release–a Helpful Adjunct?

There is no question that the most common way for most people to take their vitamins is indeed the worst way! Namely, throwing down one's vitamins first thing in the morning with hostility is the basis for the oft-heard comment that "taking vitamins will give you expensive urine!." The fact of the matter is that this is one of those many half-truths. True, taking vitamins that way will indeed produce expensive urine. Hence, it is for that very reason that there have been attempts, through the years, to put medicaments in general, and for our purposes vitamins in particular, into time- or sustained-release form.

We were very fortunate to participate in one of the first studies with time-release vitamins which we published as "Effect of Sustained Release Versus Regular Multivitamin Supplementation upon Vitamin C State" in the International Journal for Vitamin Research (39: #4, 407-415, 1969).

The general effort has been to develop delayed time-release principles with the assumption that longer intestinal transit would result in increased absorption. Our particular studies were published in 1969 and dealt with the "Spansule" product which consisted of a core of sugar and starch to which a vitamin was applied. This then was surrounded by a semipermeable coating. The coatings were tailor-made blends of selected waxes and fats whose precise composition was dictated by the physiochemical characteristics of the particular substance to be delivered. Moisture permeated the coating by osmosis and the core became swollen, eventually rupturing the coating. The phenomenon of sustained release was based on the rate of moisture permeation into hundreds of pellets with coatings of various thicknesses. The thinner coatings were found to be more permeable and ruptured first, while the thicker coatings which were progressively less permeable, were delayed in their time of rupture.

This particular experiment consisted of an examination of a regular, meaning nontime-release, versus

68

sustained-release multivitamin supplement on two measures of vitamin C in 50 presumably healthy subjects. Specifically, the study was intended to show changes in blood as determined by the plasma ascorbic acid level and in tissues as measured by the lingual ascorbic acid test time.

Actually, 50 allegedly healthy students participated in a double-blind crossover study in which vitamin C state (as measured in the blood and tissues) was evaluated before and following the administration of a multivitamin supplement in a regular versus sustained-release form.

Figure 22.1

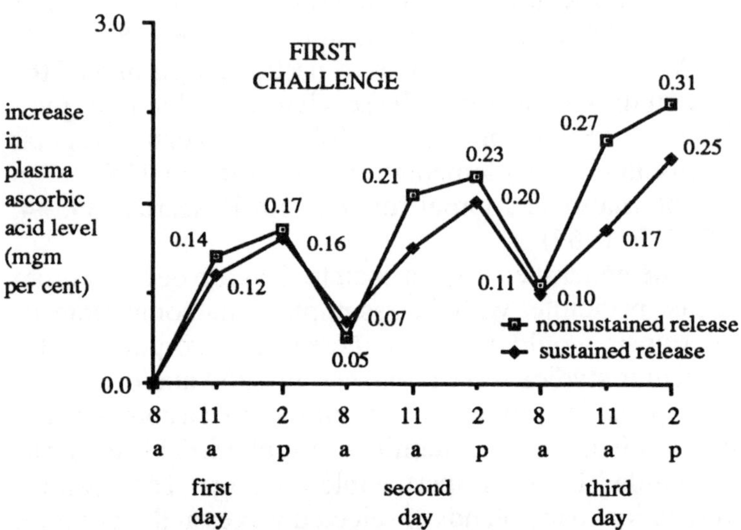

Figure 22.1 and 22.2 summarize the blood results. Initially, by random selection, one-half of the subjects, namely 25, were given a nonsustained-release vitamin supplement and the remaining 25 were provided with a sustained-release preparation. The initial challenge was three consecutive days. Both groups were given instructions to abstain from any other nutritional supplements or citrus fruit or juice intake for two days prior to this period Each subject was instructed not to eat or drink anything except water after 8:00 P.M. on the evening before the initial period and to eat only between the hours of

2:00 P.M. and 8:00 P.M. on the three test days. This allowed a daily 12-hour fasting blood sample at 8:00 A.M. and a 15-hour fasting sample at 11:00 A.M. and an 18-hour fasting sample at 2:00 P.M.

Following the initial three days of the vitamin challenge, a 13-day intermission was put into effect. Normal eating habits were allowed but abstention from vitamin supplements was continued. Restriction of citrus fruit or juice intake was reinstituted during the last two intermission days. Fasting and eating instructions were given as in the initial period. During the next three days, each

Figure 22.2

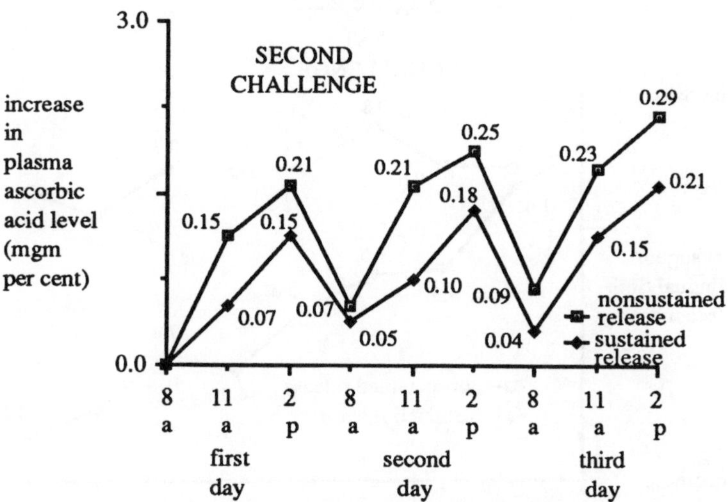

group received the supplement previously administered to the other group. Each participant was given under supervision the appropriate supplement immediately after the 8:00 A.M. blood sample was drawn. The dose was one capsule per day during both periods.

Figures 22.1 and 22.2 provide the blood conclusions. There is a statistically significant difference (p<0.005) between the formulations with the nonsustained release giving the higher plasma ascorbic acid levels than the sustained release. Parenthetic mention should be made that the order of receiving formulations (i.e. first challenge or second challenge period) showed no significant effect upon the plasma vitamin C levels. The increase in plasma ascorbic acid level over the three days and within each day are all highly statistically significantly different (p<0.001).

An examination of the tissue levels is outlined in Figures 22.3 and 22.4. The difference between formulations is highly significant (p<0.001) with the sustained release providing much lower average lingual vitamin C test times than the nonsustained release. This obviously suggests a greater delivery into the tissues with the sustained-release preparation. Secondly, the order of receiving the formulation (i.e. first challenge period or second

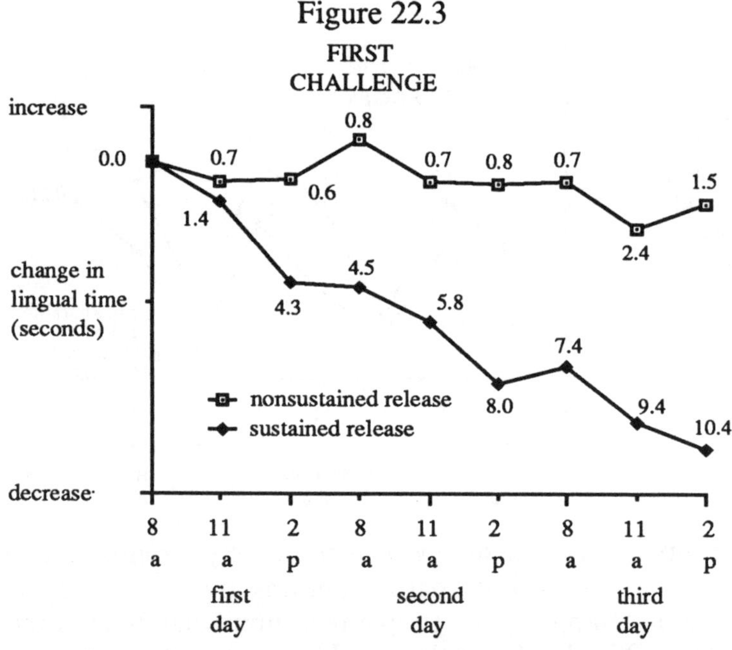

Figure 22.3

challenge period) showed no significant effect upon the lingual times. However, the analysis indicates that the comparison between formulations is not the same for the two challenge periods. In other words, there is indeed a significant interaction between the formulation and the challenge period. This is especially noted from Figures 22.3 and 22.4. Whereas the sustained release gives much lower lingual times than the nonsustained release as demonstrated in the first challenge period, the difference is much less marked in the second challenge period. Finally, the decrease in lingual time over the three days of each challenge period and over the three sampling times within each day are all highly statistically significant (p<0.001) which is also apparent from this last illustration.

Figure 22.4

SECOND
CHALLENGE

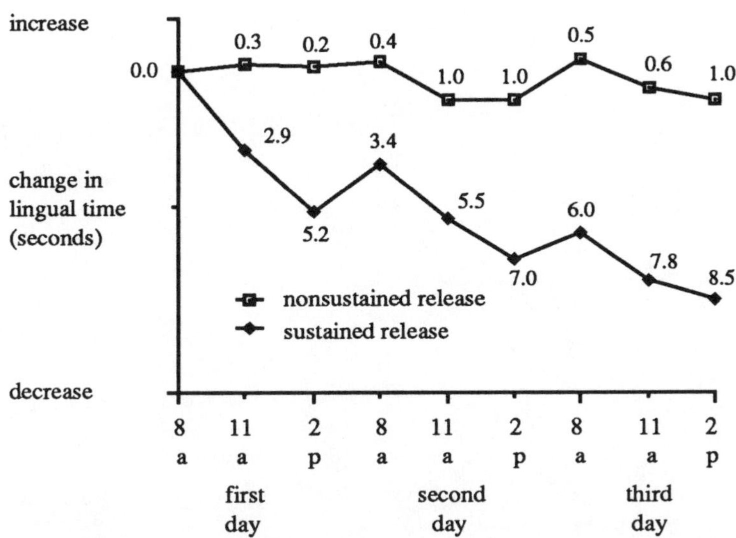

Hence, an analysis of the results suggest beyond question that the sustained-released multivitamin formulation enables greater amounts of vitamin C to reach the tissues than the nonsustained-release preparation.

PART

FOUR

VITAMIN

C

IN

ORAL

HEALTH

AND

DISEASE

Discovery consists in seeing what everybody else has seen and thinking what nobody has thought.

Albert Szent-Gyorgyi

23. Can One Demonstrate Changes in Gingival Hue by Means of Simple Orange Juice Supplementation?

At the time we attempted an answer to this question, the general consensus in dentistry (and regrettably it has not materially changed even at this time) was that vitamin C contributed very little if at all to the periodontal state. In this investigation, which we published under the title "Gingival Hue and Orange Juice" and which was released in the Journal of Dental Medicine (18: #4, 171-174, October 1963), we studied 53 presumably healthy dental students with a mean age of 27 who volunteered for this particular project. Before any studies were made, the students were divided into an experimental (to be supplemented with orange juice on a daily basis) and a control (non-supplemented) group of 27 and 26 subjects respectively. Incidentally, the choice of the group was self-elected. Each student was then given a complete oral examination. This included a study of the labial papillary and marginal gingiva of the upper and lower anterior teeth which were individually graded as zero (pink), one for slightly red, and two for moderately to severely inflamed.

The scores were calculated for the separate areas and a mean derived. Following the collection of the initial data and throughout the subsequent twelve-month period, each participant in the supplemented group was instructed to drink 8 ounces of a standardized orange juice each morning before breakfast. The juice was issued each week in a concentrated form and diluted to specifications by the students. The participants were supervised carefully to ensure cooperation in the procedure. As far as we could determine, except for the additional orange juice, there was no change in the normal daily diet of each participant.

In contrast, the nonsupplemented (control) group was instructed specifically to refrain from consuming any form of citrus fruit. This was reemphasized at frequent intervals during the experimental year.

On a mean basis, the gingival hue in the supplemented group decreased from 0.52 to 0.22; in contrast, in the nonsupplemented group, the mean increased from 0.38 to 0.73. Hence, the gingival color in the nonsupplemented group significantly worsened during the experimental one-year period. In contrast, a significant improvement in gingival hue was observed in the supplemented group.

This question obviously addresses one of the simplest and nonspecific measures of periodontal health and sickness. Other studies, listed elsewhere in this monograph, direct attention to specific periodontal problems and the possible connection of those parameters to vitamin C.

24. What about Vitamin C and Subclinical Scurvy?

There is no question but that the literature is replete with descriptions of **clinical** scurvy. Characteristically, the teeth become loose and exfoliate in the classically scorbutic patient. There is also agreement that **classical** scurvy is indeed rare. In contrast, only fragmentary information is available regarding so-called **subclinical** scurvy. Quite apart, there is considerable data available regarding clinical tooth mobility. Far less information can be obtained in connection with **subclinical** tooth mobility.

There was at the time we became interested in this problem no reported study of the relationship or lack of correlation between **subclinical** scurvy and **subclinical** tooth mobility. For that reason, we performed a study of four clinically healthy subjects over a four-month period in terms of **subclinical** ascorbic acid status and **subclinical** tooth mobility. This was subsequently published as "Subclinical Scurvy and Subclinical Tooth Mobility" in the Journal of the Western Society of Periodontology (7: #1, 6-28, March 1959).

The four subjects had a number of characteristics in common and certain dimensions that were different. For example, two of the subjects showed neither clinical nor laboratory evidence of an ascorbic acid deficiency. These same two subjects demonstrated a physiologic range of subclinical tooth mobility. The other two subjects showed no **clinical** evidence of a vitamin C deficiency but did demonstrate **laboratory** proof of a **subclinical** ascorbic acid deficiency. These two subjects differed additionally in that one had undergone orthodontic therapy during adulthood.

Initially, the subject without orthodontic treatment demonstrated teeth with only small ranges of subclinical tooth mobility (and without any clinical evidence of loose teeth). After one week of a relatively massive ascorbic acid regime, the teeth actually "loosened" and the range approached that of the two healthy subjects.

The subject with orthodontic treatment had teeth with a large range of subclinical tooth mobility initially. After two weeks on a massive ascorbic acid regime, the teeth "tightened" and the range approached that of the healthy subjects.

When vitamin therapy was discontinued, the vitamin C levels appeared to return to their original values in the last two subjects. Interestingly enough, the subclinical tooth mobility trend also seemed to suggest that their patterns were reversing to that observed at the beginning of the experiment.

Hence, within the limits of this modest experiment, there does indeed appear to be a very definite relationship between **subclinical** tooth mobility, as one measure of **subclinical** scurvy, and vitamin C state.

The subject of more obvious clinical tooth mobility and vitamin C nutriture is discussed elsewhere in this monograph.

25. Is there any Correlation Between Blood and/or Tissue Vitamin C State and Clinical Tooth Mobility?

There is no question that more teeth are lost because of periodontal reasons than tooth decay. There is also no question but that increasing clinical tooth mobility is one of most common reasons for losing teeth. Accordingly, we thought it wise to look into this problem as it relates to dietary state and actually made an attempt to solve this issue in a study of 102 subjects. This eventuated in a report entitled "A Lingual Vitamin C Test: X. Relationship to Tooth Mobility" which appeared in the International Journal for Vitamin Research (38: #3/4, 433-437, 1968).

Figure 25.1

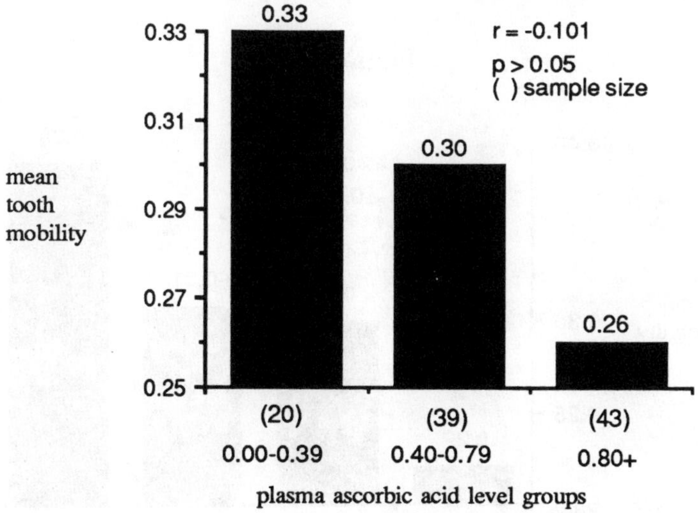

Actually, the participants were studied in terms of vitamin C state as measured under fasting conditions by means of blood (plasma ascorbic acid concentration) and tissue (lingual vitamin C test time). Specifically, tooth mobility was separately graded in each of the twelve

80

anterior teeth on a three-point scale with 0 equals no clinical tooth mobility, 1 for clinical tooth mobility less than one millimeter and 2 for clinical tooth mobility more than one millimeter. From these measurements, the mean was determined and expressed to two decimals.

Figure 25.1 depicts the relationship between plasma ascorbic acid concentration on the horizontal axis and mean clinical tooth mobility scores on the vertical dimension. It is noteworthy that those 20 subjects with the lowest and presumably the poorest vitamin C levels in the blood are associated with the greatest mean tooth mobility (0.33). Conversely, the 43 subjects with the least tooth mobility show the highest vitamin C levels in the blood (0.80+ mg. percent). Finally, those assuming an intermediate position in terms of clinical tooth mobility also assume an intermediate position in terms of vitamin C state. Notwithstanding, the overall relationship is clearly shown not to be statistically significant as judged by an r=-0.101, p>0.05.

Figure 25.2

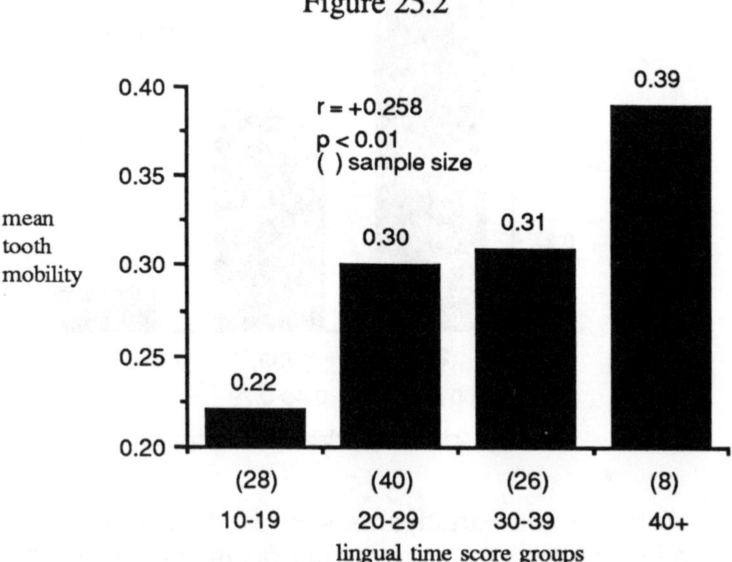

In contrast, Figure 25.2 illustrates the relationship of the lingual time, on the x-axis and mean clinical tooth mobility on the vertical axis. It is abundantly clear that there is indeed a statistically significant positive correlation ($r = +0.258$, $p<0.01$), suggesting, as the lingual time goes up (meaning relatively poorer vitamin C state), clinical tooth mobility increases.

Hence, the suggested evidence here is that while blood may not be a reflector of vitamin C state in terms of clinical tooth mobility, it seems tissue vitamin C state might well be.

This is one of a number of studies which we have performed over these many years which underlines the relative merits of examining vitamin C nutriture in the blood versus in the tissues.

26.   Can One Relate Blood Ascorbic Acid Levels to Sulcus Depth?

Sulcus or pocket depth is one of the more measurable expressions of periodontal disease. For this and other reasons, we thought it wise to look into the relationship of vitamin C nutriture to this measure of periodontal health and sickness.

This particular study included 102 subjects in which venous blood was drawn under fasting conditions and the plasma ascorbic acid concentration ascertained. Additionally, sulcus depth was measured to the nearest millimeter on the distal, mesial, labial, and lingual sides of the twelve anterior teeth. From these measurements, the mean sulcus depth was derived and was expressed to two decimal places.

Figure 26.1

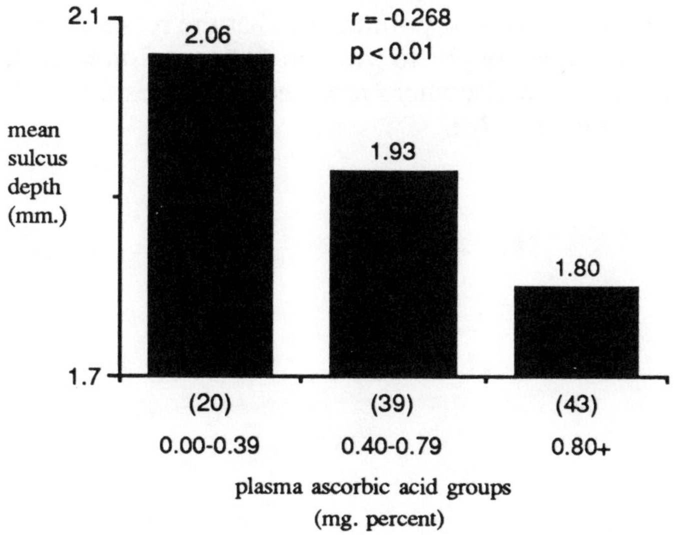

The accompanying illustration (Figure 26.1) correlates the plasma ascorbic acid levels depicted on the x-axis and the mean sulcus depth scores expressed in millimeters to the second decimal place on the ordinate. It is clear those 20 subjects with the lowest (and therefore the poorest) vitamin C levels in the plasma are characterized by those with the deepest sulci (with a mean of 2.06 millimeters). Conversely, those with the highest (and presumably the best) blood vitamin C levels (0.80+ mg. percent) parallel those with the shallowest sulcus depth (mean = 1.80 mm.). Finally, those assuming an intermediate position in terms of vitamin C state also assume an intermediate place in terms of sulcus depth.

The significance of these relationships is heightened by a statistically significant correlation (r=-0.268, p<0.01).

Hence, to the extent that one can draw conclusions from such parallelisms, the evidence seems clear that there may well be a significant negative correlation between plasma ascorbic acid concentration and mean sulcus depth. These have been stated in the paper "A Lingual Vitamin C Test: XI. Relationship to Gingival Sulcus Depth" which appeared in the International Journal for Vitamin Research (38: #5, 512-516, 1968).

It also should be pointed out that the relationship of gingival sulcus depth to vitamin C as measured in the tissue has been elsewhere reported (see Question 27 beginning on page 85).

27. Can One Connect Tissue Vitamin C State to Sulcus Depth?

Because of the great importance of sulcus depth in periodontal health and sickness, vitamin C state has been studied very carefully both in the blood and in the tissues.

This is the story of 102 subjects who participated in a rather extensive experiment in which a number of oral parameters and vitamin C state were employed.

Figure 27.1

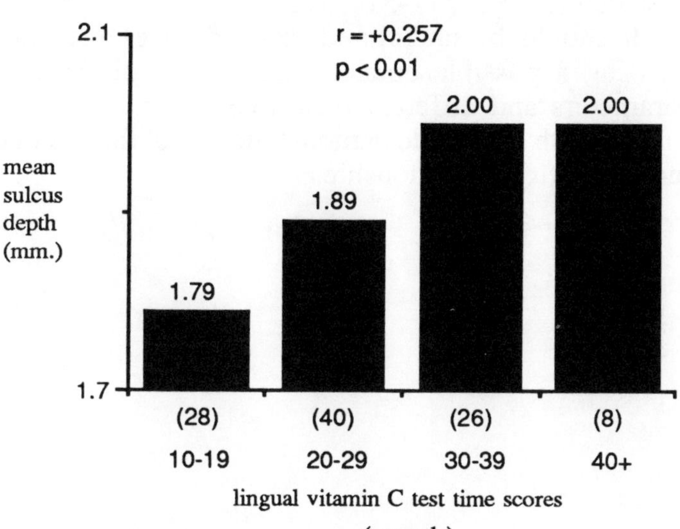

In this particular portion of the study, the lingual vitamin C test was measured under fasting conditions. Sulcus depth was ascertained to the nearest millimeter on the distal, mesial, labial, and lingual sides of the twelve anterior teeth. The mean sulcus depth so derived from these 48 measurements was expressed to the second decimal.

The illustration (Figure 27.1) shows the relationship between lingual time described on the horizontal axis and the mean sulcus depth pictured on the vertical dimension.

Interestingly, those with the shortest lingual time (suggesting the best vitamin C state) in a range of 10 to 19 seconds show the shallowest sulcus depth (actually with a mean of 1.79 mm). Conversely, those 26 plus 8 subjects with the longest lingual time (30+ seconds) are accompanied by the deepest sulci with a mean of 2.00 mm. The other group with an intermediate lingual test time demonstrates an intermediate sulcus depth score. The significance of this positive correlation is clearly shown by an $r = +0.257$ and a $p<0.01$.

This material was published in an article entitled "A Lingual Vitamin C Test: XI. Relationship to Gingival Sulcus Depth" in the International Journal for Vitamin Research (38: #5, 512-516, 1968).

It should be underlined that, of all of the studies showing a possible connection between different oral parameters and different measures of vitamin C state, sulcus depth appears to demonstrate one of the, if not the, most significant relationships.

28. Of What Possible Importance Might Vitamin C be in Alveolar Bone Loss?

One of the most sensitive measures of periodontal health and sickness is the presence or absence of alveolar bone loss. However, what we saw in earlier experiments were correlations and not cause and effect studies. Naturally, we wished more information regarding the causative role of vitamin C in alveolar bone loss and we put together a report entitled "Ascorbic Acid and Alveolar Bone Loss" which appeared in Oral Surgery, Oral Medicine, and Oral Pathology (15: #5, 555-565, May 1962).

In this investigation of the relationship of ascorbic acid to alveolar bone loss, fifty-four dental students (with a mean age of 27 years) were selected on a voluntary basis. Before any examinations were made, the students were divided into an experimental and a control group of equal numbers on a completely arbitrary system by means of self-selection. Each student was then given a complete oral examination.

Following the collection of the initial data and throughout the subsequent twelve-month period, each participant in the experimental group (to be referred to hereafter as the supplemented group) was instructed to drink 8 ounces of a standardized orange juice each morning before breakfast. The participants were supervised very carefully to ensure cooperation in the procedure. Except for the additional intake of the 8 ounces of orange juice per day, there was to be no change in the normal daily diet in any of the group.

In contrast to the supplemented group, the control group (to be referred to hereafter as the nonsupplemented group) was instructed specifically to refrain from consuming citrus fruit in order to validate the experimental procedure. This was reemphasized at frequent intervals during the subsequent experimental year. Except for the elimination of citrus fruits in any form from the diet, no attempt was made to alter the normal daily dietary habits. At the end of the experimental twelve-month period, each dental student was recalled and submitted to a re-examination of the oral structures, both clinically and roentgenographically, as in the initial procedures.

An impartial examiner was selected to perform the measurements of alveolar bone loss. These measurements were made with a specially constructed transparent ruler on which ten radii were marked, each equidistant from the margin of the plastic strip, thus allowing for the so-called normal distance of the alveolar crest to the cementoenamel junction. To obtain the measurement, the roentgenograms were placed on an illuminated board. The ruler was positioned on top of the roentgenograms so that the upper margin coincided with the interproximal cementoenamel junction and the last radius was superimposed over the apex of the tooth being measured. This procedure allowed the examiner to observe the height of the alveolar crest (in percentage) through the ruler and to determine whether the alveolar crests were on or between two radii. The measurements were obtained to the nearest 5 percent.

Measurements were made in this manner for both the mesial and the distal interproximal surfaces of the lower central and lateral incisors. This area was chosen because (1) all subjects possessed lower anterior teeth and (2) roentgenographic distortion could be minimized.

A study of the results (Figure 28.1) disclosed that the group without supplementation decreased 1.5 percent during the experimental year (93.8 to 92.3 percent); whereas, the supplemented group declined 1.2 percent during the same period (94.4 to 93.2 percent). Thus, for the moment, it appeared that there had been a slightly greater alveolar bone loss (actually 0.3 percent) in the nonsupplemented group than in the supplemented group. However, there were no statistically significant differences in any of the conditions studied.

It is evident that, from these available data, one cannot conclude any cause-and-effect relationship between ascorbic acid intake and alveolar bone loss. It is, of course, possible that such a relationship does indeed not exist. On the other hand, there is the possibility that the samples were too small for true differences to be detected. Also, there is the possibility that the time factor may be a variable which had not been given sufficient consideration. In other words, it is conceivable that there does, indeed, exist a relationship between ascorbic acid and alveolar bone loss but that a period of more than one year is required to demonstrate evidence of this relationship. The possiblity indicates the need for a longitudinal study.

Such an investigation was not, at that time, possible. However, it was thought interesting to extrapolate and see what the alveolar bone height patterns would be for the 27-year-old students if they were to continue as they had for the one-year period.

Figure 28.1 shows the findings at the start of the

Figure 28.1

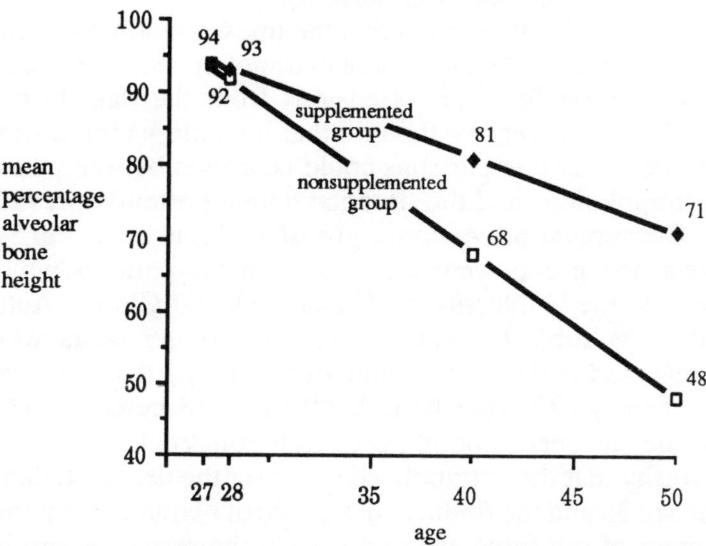

experiment. In whole numbers, both the supplemented and also nonsupplemented groups showed a mean percentage alveolar bone loss of 6 percent (alveolar bone height, 94 percent). One year later, the supplemented group lost 1 percent in alveolar bone height (from 94 to 93 percent), while the alveolar bone height in the nonsupplemented group was reduced by approximately 2 percent (from 94 to 92 percent).

In Figure 28.1 these lines have been extended to age 50. Since no other information was available, it was assumed that the patterns would continue in a linear fashion. This assumption obviously can be questioned. However, assuming such a pattern to be correct, one might estimate that, at age 40, the supplemented group would have approximately 81 percent alveolar bone height in contrast to approximately 68 percent for the nonsupplemented group. In other words, there might conceivably be a difference, at age 40, of 13 percent more alveolar bone loss in the nonsupplemented group than in the supplemented group. Extending these extrapolations to age 50, one notes that the supplemented group might have lost approximately 29 percent of bone height, whereas the nonsupplemented group might now be without more than one-half of the bone (52 percent).

It should be recalled that the lines extending beyond age 28 (Figure 28.1) are pure extrapolations. There is no justification for such extensions from the data in this study. However, we thought that it would be interesting to see if any comparisons could be drawn between these extrapolations and the situation which presently prevails in the population. Accordingly, 46 males in the 25- to 54-year age group were selected from the patients which visited the University of Alabama Dental Clinic. Actually, 33 subjects, with a mean age of 35 years were measured in this experiment. It was found that the mean percentage alveolar bone height was 78 percent. This value has been superimposed in Figure 28.2. It is noteworthy that the extrapolated value for the dental students at age 35 and the findings in a group of dental clinic population of the same age is precisely the same. A similar estimate was made at age 40. Again, the difference between the extrapolations of the data for the dental students and the actual findings of the selected population was only 5 percent (68 versus 63 percent). Finally, a similar comparison at age 45 revealed that the two values varied by only 1 percent (57 versus 58 percent).

These observations are not intended to replace a

much-needed longitudinal study. However, they seem to indicate that the extrapolated line may be more real than imaginary and that young dental students without vitamin supplementation might sometime later (with regard to alveolar bone loss, at least) be somewhat similar to the patients who were used to establish the estimates of alveolar bone height in later years.

Unfortunately, there are no studies to which one can refer to verify the extrapolated lines for those students who received vitamin C supplementation. However, information was available in the laboratory of the Section on Oral Medicine at the University of Alabama School of Dentistry, regarding plasma ascorbic acid levels and alveolar bone height in 170 dental patients. Those of the 170 with plasma ascorbic acid levels greater than 0.9 mg. percent (73 persons) were put in one group. This was done

Figure 28.2

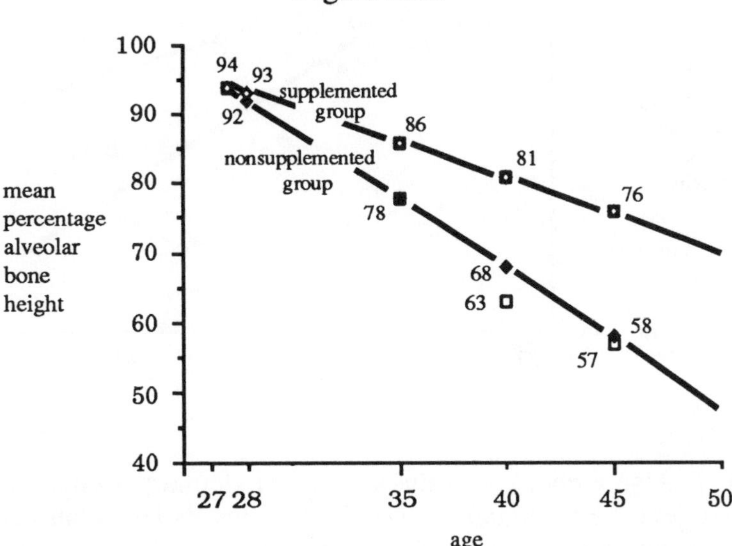

because this level of vitamin C is well within physiologic limits according to most investigators. The mean alveolar bone height for the subjects at ages 35, 40 and 45 were determined for the group with acceptable plasma levels. It is noteworthy that the scores obtained closely approximate those of the extrapolated line for the dental students who received vitamin C supplementation (Figure 28.3). For example, the extrapolated line at age 35 indicates alveolar bone height of about 86 percent. Figure 28.3 also reveals that the dental patients with plasma levels greater than 0.9 mg. percent averaged 87 percent alveolar bone height (a difference of 1 percent). Also shown are differences of 3 percent and 6 percent at ages 40 and 45. Thus, on the average, alveolar bone loss in patients with relatively good plasma ascorbic acid levels is quite similar to the extrapolations for dental students under vitamin C supplemented conditions.

Figure 28.3

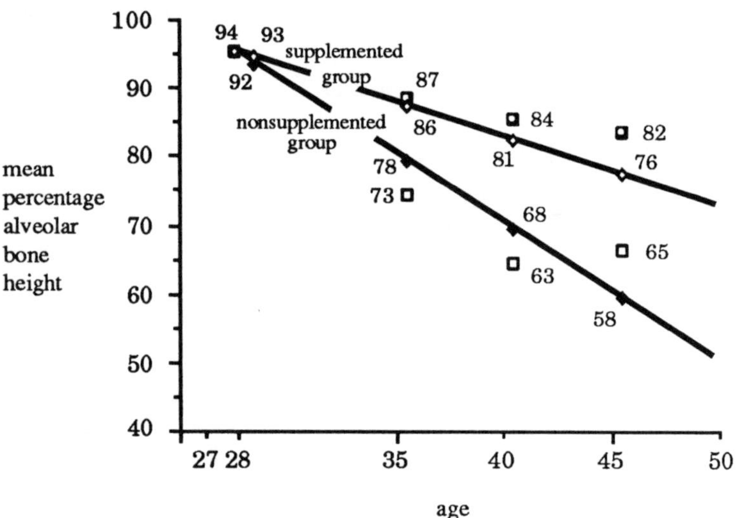

Also a check was made of those dental patients (90 subjects) with plasma ascorbic acid levels less than 0.1 mg. percent. This level is generally regarded as being indicative of poor ascorbic acid intake. It should be noted that these points closely approximate the extrapolated line for the group of nonsupplemented dental students. For example, at age 35 the prediction for the students is that alveolar bone height will be 73 percent. This group of dental patients yielded a 78 percent (a difference of 5 percent). Likewise, differences at 40 and 45 years proved to be 5 and 7 percent respectively.

While this experiment does not conclude without question that ascorbic acid and alveolar bone loss are indeed significantly related, it does provide very interesting results highly suggestive of such a cause-and-effect correlation.

29.   What About a Connection Between Oral Hygiene and Vitamin C Tissue State?

There is no question of the importance of oral hygiene in dental health and sickness. Strangely, practically little

Table 29.1

oral hygiene evaluation

0 = No debris was collected
1 = A small amount of debris equal in size to an explorer point
2 = An amount twice the size of explorer point
3 = An amount which could be picked off as a plaque or pellicle
4 = The whole buccal surface of the tooth covered with debris

has been considered to demonstrate the importance (or unimportance) of vitamin C state in oral hygiene.

Figure 29.1

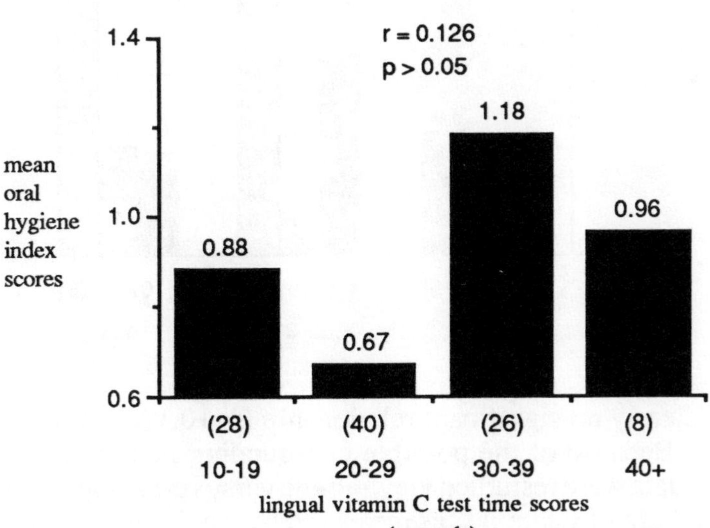

One hundred two subjects shared in this experiment.

The lingual vitamin C test was measured under fasting conditions. Oral hygiene was graded on a five-point scale (Table 29.1) with zero indicating the best possible oral hygiene score and five the worst. The grades for the twelve anterior teeth were added and a mean oral hygiene score derived from these measurements was expressed to two decimals. This material was collected and appeared as "A Lingual Vitamin C Test: XIII. Relationship to Oral Hygiene" which appeared in the International Journal for Vitamin Research (38: #5, 524-530, 1968).

Figure 29.1 pictorially portrays the relationship of lingual vitamin C test scores on the horizontal axis and the mean oral hygiene scores on the vertical dimension. There

Figure 29.2

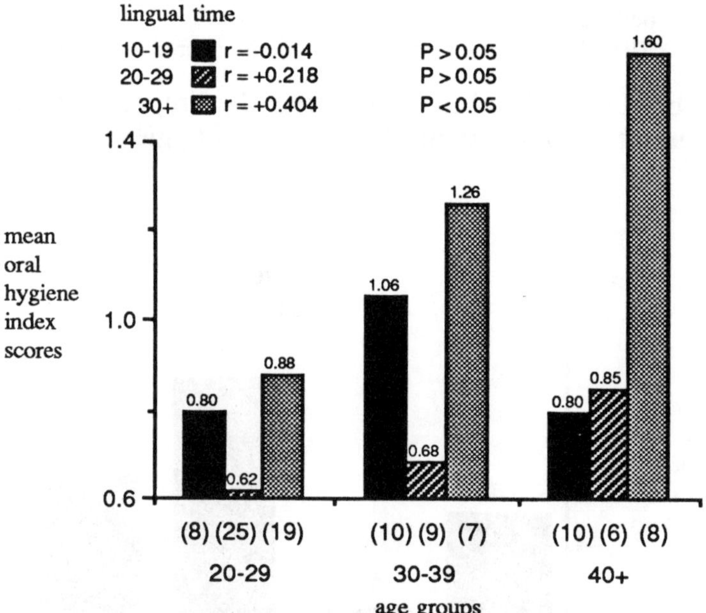

is clearly no significant relationship (r=+0.126, p>0.05).

Because of the possible confounding nature of age, the data were restudied viewing age versus oral hygiene in the light of vitamin C as measured by the lingual vitamin C Test. The illustration (Figure 29.2) shows age on the x-axis and the mean oral hygiene scores on the y-axis.

There is only a statistically significant relationship between age and oral hygiene in the group with the poorest vitamin C test time (30+ seconds) demonstrated by the stippled columns. This is underscored by an r=+0.404, and a p<0.05.

Hence, within the limits of this study, there seems to be a connection between oral hygiene and vitamin C state as measured by the vitamin C tissue test. Specifically, as vitamin C state becomes poorer, oral hygiene increases.

30. What About a Possible Relationship Between Blood Vitamin C and Oral Hygiene?

In the final analysis, there are a number of oral factors which have been blamed for possible periodontal disease. These are variously named and variously blamed. In general, the overall designation for local irritating factors in the genesis of periodontal pathosis is oral hygiene. Hence, consideration has been given to an analysis of the possible relationship between blood vitamin C concentration and oral hygiene. This appeared in a document entitled "A Lingual Vitamin C Test: XIII. Relationship to Oral Hygiene" which was published in the International Journal for Vitamin Research (38: #5, 524-530, 1968).

This is a study of 102 presumably healthy subjects. Venous blood was drawn under fasting conditions and plasma ascorbic acid concentration was ascertained. Additionally, oral hygiene was graded on a five-point scale as shown in the accompanying table (Table 30.1). The scores for the twelve anterior teeth were summed and a mean oral hygiene score derived from those measurements expressed to two decimals.

Table 30.1

oral hygiene evaluation

0 = No debris was collected
1 = A small amount of debris equal in size to an explorer point
2 = An amount twice the size of explorer point
3 = An amount which could be picked off as a plaque or pellicle
4 = The whole buccal surface of the tooth covered with debris

A study of plasma ascorbic acid levels in terms of oral hygiene values is pictorially portrayed in Figure 30.1. On a mean basis it appears that the poorest oral hygiene (1.02) is associated in the subjects with the poorest plasma vitamin C level (0.00 - 0.39 mg. percent). Conversely, those with the best oral hygiene (0.76) parallel those with the highest plasma vitamin C level (0.80+ mg. percent). Those with the intermediate scores fit in appropriately.

Figure 30.1

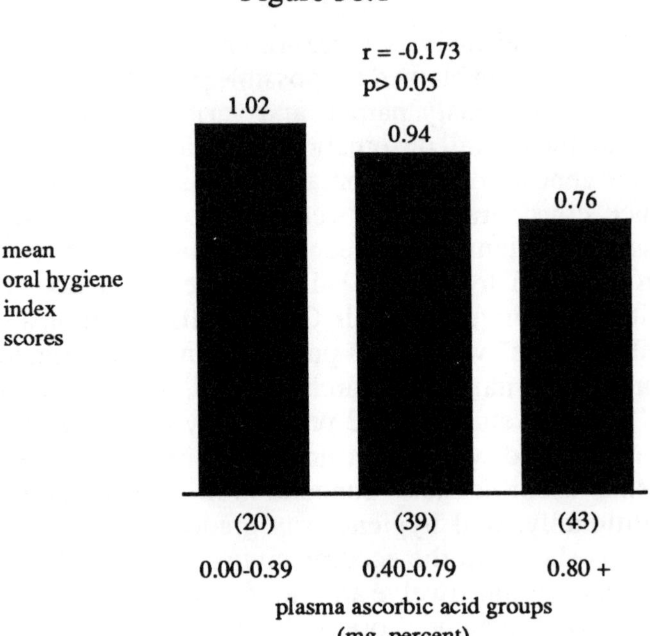

However, a statistical analysis does not suggest a significant relationship (r = -0.173, p >0.05).

Because age may possibly play a complicating factor, the data were restudied viewing age versus oral hygiene in the light of plasma ascorbic acid levels. Figure 30.2 shows the age groups displayed on the abscissa and mean oral hygiene scores on the ordinate. More specifically, as plasma ascorbic acid level increases, oral hygiene decreases. Thus, in the six subjects with the poorest vitamin C level (0.00-0.39 mg. percent), the oral hygiene score is the highest (1.21). Conversely, in the 13 subjects with the highest plasma ascorbic acid level (0.80+ mg. percent), there is the lowest oral hygiene score (1.00). Finally, those occupying an intermediate position in terms of plasma ascorbic acid level (0.40-0.79) show the intermediate oral hygiene score of 1.12 in the remaining five subjects. Additionally, the point should be made that these relationships are indeed statistically significant (r = +0.365, p<0.05).

Figure 30.2

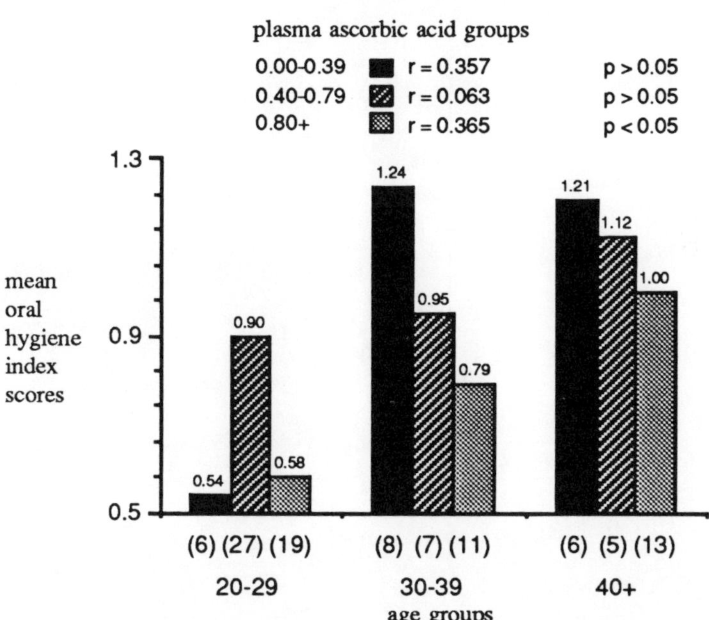

Parenthetic mention should be made that this very same relationship has been demonstrated between oral hygiene and tissue vitamin C state elsewhere (p.95).

31. Is There a Known Connection Between Oral Tartar (Calculus) and Tissue Vitamin C State?

The importance of calculus in the genesis of oral disease is much discussed. Surprisingly, there is practically

Table 31.1

calculus scoring

0 = No calculus present.
1 = Supragingival calculus covering no more than one-third of exposed tooth surface.
2 = Supragingival calculus covering more than one-third but not more than two-thirds of the exposed tooth surface or the presence of individual flecks of subgingival calculus around the cervical of the tooth or both.
3 = Supragingival calculus covering more than two-thirds of exposed tooth surface or a continuous heavy band of subgingival calculus around the cervical portion of the tooth or both.

Figure 31.1

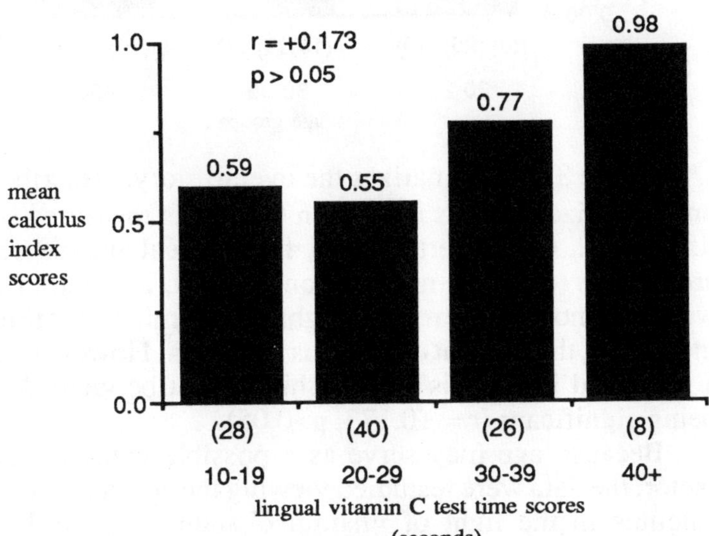

nothing in the literature on the possible role of vitamin C in the causation of oral tartar.

It is for that very reason that an attempt was made to answer this question by studying 102 presumably healthy subjects who were graded in terms of calculus on a four-point scale. Table 31.1 outlines the grading system for tartar. Additionally, the lingual vitamin C test was performed as a measure of ascorbic acid status.

Figure 31.2

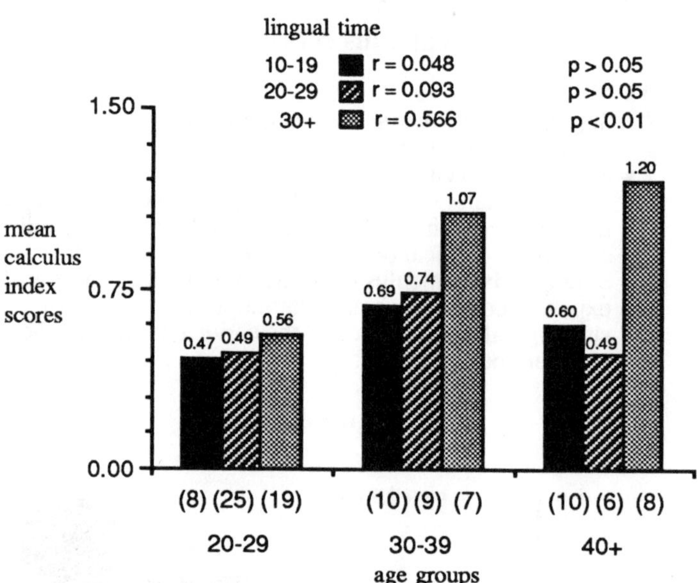

Figure 31.1 summarizes the overall story. Described on the horizontal axis is vitamin C state as measured by tissue level. On the vertical axis, the mean calculus scores are shown. There is no question but that, as vitamin C worsens (moving from left to right the vitamin C test time increases), the amount of calculus increases. However, on a statistical basis, this relationship cannot be viewed as being significant (r = +0.173, p>0.05).

Because age may serve as a possible confounding factor, the data were restudied viewing the age versus oral calculus in the light of vitamin C state. Figure 31.2 compares the age on the horizontal axis and mean total calculus scores on the vertical dimension. It is abundantly clear that there is only a statistically significant relationship between age and oral calculus in the group with the poorest vitamin C test time (30+ seconds). This is underscored by an $r = +0.566$ and a $p<0.01$.

Hence, within the limits of this study, there does indeed appear to be at least in subset analysis, a significant relationship between tartar on the teeth and the vitamin C tissue state.

This unusual experiment obviously needs more study and clarification. However, what we do know was described in "A Lingual Vitamin C Test: XIV. Relationship to Oral Calculus" which appeared in the International Journal for Vitamin Research (38: #5, 531-537, 1968).

32. What Demonstrated Connection Can One Show Between Tartar on the Teeth and Blood Vitamin C Level?

It is generally held in traditional dental circles that tartar on the teeth (calculus) is the result of poor oral hygiene (meaning poor oral care) stemming from a poor art of cleansing. Additionally, it is recognized that calculus is one of the important factors in the genesis of periodontal disease.

Accordingly, we thought it would be interesting to examine the possible relationship between tartar on the teeth and the blood vitamin C concentration. This relationship was reported in a paper entitled "A Lingual Vitamin C Test: XIV. Relationship to Oral Calculus" which was published in the International Journal for Vitamin Research (38: #5, 531-537, 1968).

Table 32.1

calculus scoring

0 = No calculus present.
1 = Supragingival calculus covering no more than one-third of exposed tooth surface.
2 = Supragingival calculus covering more than one-third but not more than two-thirds of the exposed tooth surface or the presence of individual flecks of subgingival calculus around the cervical of the tooth or both.
3 = Supragingival calculus covering more than two-thirds of exposed tooth surface or a continuous heavy band of subgingival calculus around the cervical portion of the tooth or both.

Actually, 102 presumably healthy subjects were examined in terms of a possible relationship between tartar on the teeth and blood vitamin C concentration. Venous blood was drawn under fasting conditions and the plasma ascorbic acid level established. Calculus was graded on a four-point scale as shown in Table 32.1.

Figure 32.1 pictorially portrays the relationship between plasma ascorbic acid levels depicted on the horizontal axis versus mean calculus scores displayed on the vertical. There is absolutely no question but that the most amount of calculus (0.96) appears in the group characterized by the lowest plasma ascorbic acid concentration (0.00-0.39 mg. percent); the least calculus (0.55) associated with those with the highest vitamin C level (0.80+ mg. percent). Finally, the intermediate group in terms of plasma level enjoys an intermediate position in terms of the amount of calculus. There is no question but that this inverse relationship is highly significant ($r = -0.273$, $p<0.01$).

Figure 32.1

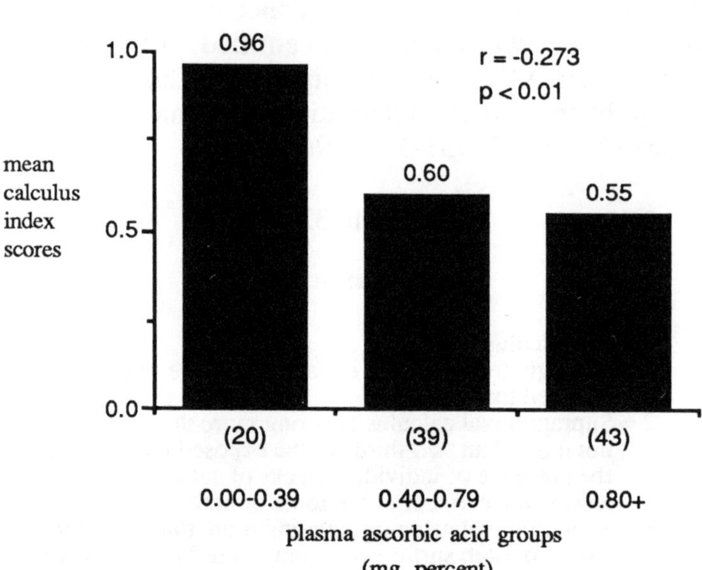

Hence, within the limits of this simple experiment, which is unknown in traditional dental circles, there seems to be a significant negative correlation between plasma ascorbic acid concentration (as one measure of vitamin C state) and the tartar (calculus) on the teeth.

It should be pointed out that we have elsewhere (p. 103) reported a study of the possible relationship between calculus and tissue vitamin C state as against blood levels shown in this experiment.

33. Is Oral Hygiene (However Defined) Related to Vitamin C State?

There is no question but that oral hygiene appears to be a significant factor in the genesis of periodontal pathosis. These very same reports disclose that the term **oral hygiene** might well have two meanings. Thus, oral hygiene signifies the state of cleanliness and the art of cleansing.

Ordinarily, the common usage of the term **oral hygiene** frequently does not recognize these differences. This likely stems from the fact that it is generally assumed that good oral hygiene (oral cleanliness) is the result of good cleansing techniques (also known as **good oral**

Figure 33.1

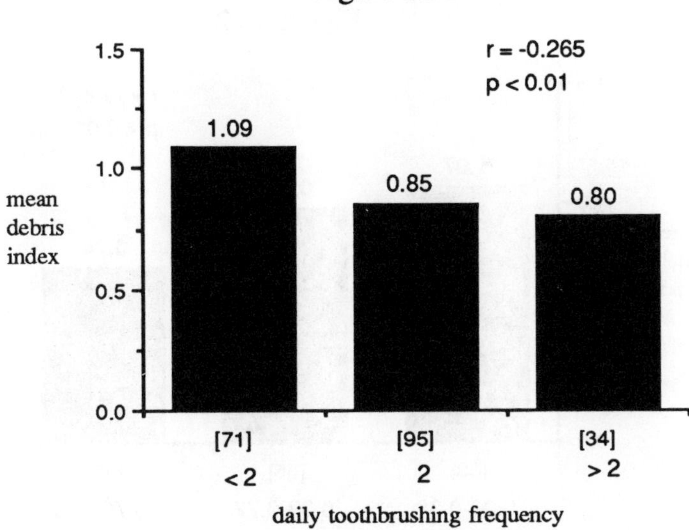

hygiene). Conversely, poor oral hygiene (**lack of oral cleanliness**) is customarily regarded as the result of ineffective tooth cleansing procedures (also known as **poor oral hygiene**). Thus, when the term oral hygiene is used, it is frequently not certain whether reference is made to tooth cleansing or tooth cleanliness.

With this in mind, we attempted to answer three very straightforward questions. First, to what extent does tooth cleanliness correlate with tooth cleansing, irrespective of host state? Secondly, to what degree does tooth cleanliness correlate with one biochemical measure of health status, the plasma ascorbic acid level, regardless of tooth cleansing? Finally, is the correlation of tooth cleansing and tooth cleanliness altered when viewed in the light of host state (plasma ascorbic acid level)?

In answer to the first question, Figure 33.1 shows that there does indeed appear to be a statistically significant inverse relationship between tooth cleansing (toothbrush frequency) and tooth cleanliness (debris score) irrespective of host state. In other words, as tooth cleansing rises, tooth cleanliness increases (r = -0.265, p<0.01).

Figure 33.2

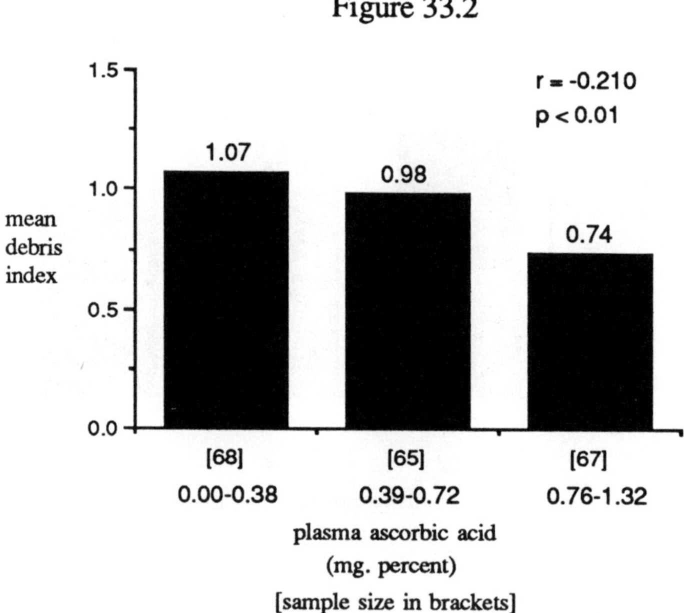

Additionally, as shown in the second illustration Figure 33.2, and within the limits of these data, there appears to be a statistically significant inverse relationship between vitamin C state and debris, irrespective of tooth cleansing habits. In other words, as vitamin C rises, tooth cleanliness rises.

Finally, as shown in Figure 33.3, the frequency of daily toothbrushing is described on the abscissa and the mean debris scores on the ordinate. Additionally, the 200 subjects were divided into two equal subgroups. The 100 subjects with the poorer plasma ascorbic acid levels (0.00 - 0.59 mg. percent) are shown by the dark columns and the other 100 with the better vitamin C state (0.60+ mg. percent) by the stippled columns. Attention is directed to

Figure 33.3

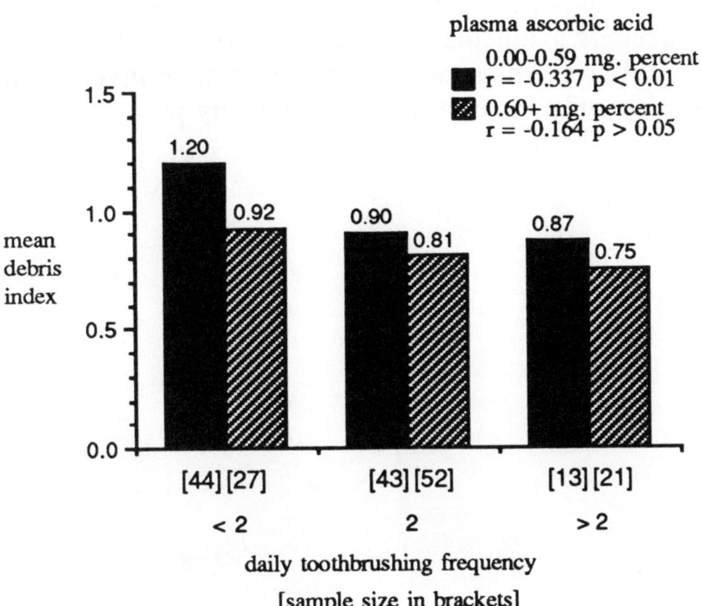

the fact that in those showing the lower plasma ascorbic acid levels, there is indeed a statistically significant inverse correlation (r = -0.337, p< 0.01) between toothbrushing and debris values. In other words, the greater the toothbrushing frequency, the less debris in subjects with relatively poor vitamin C state. It is particularly noteworthy that this correlation (r = -0.337) is higher than the correlation between toothbrushing and debris (r = -0.265), irrespective of vitamin C state and the correlation between plasma ascorbic acid level and debris ($r = -0.210$), irrespective of tooth cleansing frequency. In contrast, no such statistically significant correlation ($r = -0.164$, $p>0.05$) prevails between toothbrushing frequency and debris in the subjects with the higher, and therefore the better, plasma ascorbic acid values.

As far as we can determine, this is the only attempt in stomatology to explain the discrepancy shown by the fact that some people need more oral hygiene (cleansing) than other individuals. This report was released as "An Ecologic Study of Oral Hygiene" in the Journal of Periodontology and Periodontics (40: #8, 476-480, August 1969).

It is important to underline that the data suggest that, with regard to the final question, toothbrushing frequency and debris correlate significantly and in an inverse relationship only in subjects with relatively poor vitamin C state.

34. Are there any Advantages in Utilizing Sustained-Release Multivitamins Including Vitamin C for the Treatment of Gingival Pathology?

There is no question but that the desired method for consuming nutrients is by diet. However, for many different reasons, some understandable if not desirable, supplementation is in order. Hence, there has been developing interest in different methods of supplementation and this has led to an investigation of time-release vitamin preparations.

This study was designed to examine the relative effect of a regular versus a sustained-release multivitamin supplement upon the gingival state of presumably healthy young men. It was released under the title "Effect of Regular versus Sustained-Release Multivitamin Supplementation upon Periodontal Parameters: I. Gingival State" which appeared in the International Journal for Vitamin Research (39: #3, 314-319, 1969).

Information was particularly sought regarding the relative effects of such preparations when subjects are initially matched according to gingival state. Finally, an attempt was made to examine the gingival results of time-release versus nontime-release preparations when viewed in terms of relatively healthy versus diseased gingiva.

In answer to the first question, there is no doubt but that greater beneficial effects are derived from sustained-release versus regular multivitamin supplementation. Specifically, the improvement was 38 percent with the time-release and 12 percent with the regular preparation.

With regard to the second question, there is also no argument but that the difference between time-release and nontime-release is greater. Whereas, in the nonmatched group the difference was approximately 300 percent, when matched the difference was about 450 percent.

Finally, the results of the group with the relatively poor gingival state suggests that there is approximately a 17 percent reduction in gingival score with the regular preparation, in contrast to a 41 percent improvement in gingival inflammation with the time-release supplement.

It should be added that this study consisted of 50 presumably healthy dental students. At the first visit, on a Tuesday, the gingiva of the four mandibular incisor teeth were graded on a four-point scale. The individual scores were summed and a mean, expressed to one decimal, derived. Immediately following grading, the group was randomly divided into two subgroups of 25 subjects each. Each student received one capsule at 7:45 A.M. on Tuesday, Wednesday and Thursday of the same week. The contents consisted of a standard multivitamin preparation. All of the capsules looked alike and were indistinguishable. However, one-half of the group on a random basis, received a regular preparation; the other one-half of the group was given a sustained-release supplement. It should be pointed out that, in both cases, the preparations contained 70 mg. of vitamin C. The gingiva was regraded by the same examiner on Friday of the same week with no knowledge of the original scores or the nature of the supplements.

There is no question but the evidence indicates that the sustained-release preparation is much more effective than the regular supplement in terms of gingival improvement.

Similarly, studies have been done with a view of examining sulcus depth and clinical tooth mobility and these experiments have been described elsewhere (p. 115).

35. Is There any Justification for Time-Release Vitamin Supplementation in Oral Health?

It is noteworthy that, almost without exception, the desirability of using time-release preparations is justified by demonstrating that, with such products, blood levels are sustained higher and longer.

At the time we were studying this problem, there was not one single report showing the **clinical** desirability, if at all, of using time-release vitamin supplements.

We looked at this problem and released several reports. This particular one is entitled "Effect of Regular versus Sustained-Release Multivitamin Supplementation upon Periodontal Parameters: II. Sulcus Depth and Clinical Tooth Mobility" which appeared in the International Journal for Vitamin Research (39: #4, 476-485, 1969).

Fifty presumably healthy dental students participated in this experiment. At the first visit (Tuesday of a week) sulcus depth on the buccal, lingual, mesial, and distal of the four mandibular incisor teeth was graded to the nearest millimeter. The sixteen individual scores were summed and a mean expressed to one decimal. Concurrently, clinical tooth mobility in the four incisor teeth was graded according to the following method: 0 = no mobility, 1 = slight mobility, 2 = mobility of approximately 1 millimeter, 3 = mobility greater than 1 millimeter. The four individuals' scores were summed and a mean expressed to one decimal derived.

Immediately following the grading, the group was randomly divided into two subgroups of 25 subjects each. Each participant received one capsule at 7:45 A.M. on Tuesday, Wednesday, and Thursday of the same week. The contents of each capsule were precisely the same, and the capsules were otherwise indistinguishable. However, one-half of the group, on a random basis, received a regular multivitamin preparation. The other group was administered the sustained time-release form of this same preparation. Both supplements contained 70 mg. of vitamin C. Sulcus depth and clinical tooth mobility were regraded by the same examiner on Friday of the same experimental week with no knowledge of the initial scores or the nature of the supplements.

In general, it can be concluded that both gingival sulcus depth and clinical tooth mobility improved more significantly with time-release than with regular supplementation. Additionally, this became more evident when the groups were matched in terms of oral health. Finally, the significance of time-release supplementation became more sharply defined in those with relatively poor sulcus depth and greater tooth mobility.

Hence, within the limits of this very unique experiment, there seems to be evidence that there is good reason, as measured clinically, for time-release vitamin C preparations.

36. Vitamin C and the Water Soluble Bioflavonoids—Are They Synergistic: A Study of Clinical Tooth Mobility?

It has long been known that the water soluble bioflavonoids and vitamin C are found, as it were, packaged together in many natural products such as oranges, limes and lemons. The so-called purists in the health field have taken this to mean that there is good reason for this combination. The more conservative scientific community has recognized the possibility of potentiation or synergism but have constantly reminded us of the paucity of supportive data. It was this confusion in the scientific literature that led us to look at the possibility of studying the relative merits, if indeed they are there, of vitamin C with and without the water soluble bioflavonoids.*

One hundred and two presumably healthy subjects participated in this experiment. The selection was a random one from volunteers at the University of Alabama Medical and Extension Centers and from the Birmingham Fire Department. Table 36.1 summarizes the age and sex distribution of the group.

Table 36.1

patient age and sex distribution

age groups	male group number	percentage	female group number	percentage	total group number	percentage
20-29	25	25.5	27	26.5	52	51.0
30-39	17	16.7	9	8.8	26	25.5
40-49	12	11.8	6	5.9	18	17.7
50-59	2	1.9	4	3.9	6	5.8
total	56	54.9	46	45.1	102	100.0

*Full particulars have been published in a paper entitled "Local and Systemic Influences in Periodontal Disease: IV. Effect of Prophylaxis and Natural Versus Synthetic Vitamin C Upon Clinical Tooth Mobility" which appeared in the International Journal of Vitamin Research (34: #2, 202-218, 1964).

All subjects reported to the Department of Oral Medicine following a 12-hour fast. Upon admission, a fasting venous blood sample was drawn. The oral examinations were all performed by the same individual with no knowledge of earlier records or therapeutic regimes.

Clinical tooth mobility grading was accomplished on a four-point scale (Table 36.2).

Table 36.2

tooth mobility scoring system

0 = no mobility.
1 = slight mobility labio-lingually.
2 = marked mobility labio-lingually plus mesiodistal mobility.
3 = extreme mobility labio-lingually and mesiodistally plus
     vertical mobility into the socket.

Following the clinical examination, by a table of random numbers, the patients were arranged into four groups. The therapeutic regimes are outlined in Table 36.3.

Table 36.3

composition of capsules

Group 1   100 mg. milk sugar per capsule.
Group 2   100 mg. synthetic vitamin C.
Group 3   100 mg. synthetic vitamin C plus 100 mg. citrus
          bioflavonoids.
Group 4   100 mg. natural vitamin C concentrate plus 100 mg.
          citrus bioflavonoids.

It should be underlined that all capsules looked exactly alike. Thus, neither the patient nor the examiner were aware at any time during the experimental period regarding the preparation employed.

At the completion of the first visit, each patient was instructed to take by mouth three capsules per day for three weeks. Thus, 25 subjects received a placebo, 25 were given a 300 mg. synthetic vitamin C daily, 25 were administered 300 mg. synthetic vitamin C plus 300 mg.

citrus bioflavonoids per day, and the remaining 27 were supplemented with 300 mg. of a natural vitamin C concentrate with 300 mg. water soluble bioflavonoids each day.

Approximately 21 days later each of the patients returned. All participants were re-examined clinically and biochemically without reference to the earlier records or the nature of the supplementation.

By this method, it was possible to evaluate the effect of four different systemic therapeutic regimes (Table 36.4).

Table 36.4

tooth mobility change after systemic therapy (unscaled side)

tooth mobility grades	natural vitamin C concentrate plus bioflavonoids		synthetic vitamin C plus bioflavonoids		synthetic vitamin C		placebo	
	initial	final	initial	final	initial	final	initial	final
0	112	138	110	134	114	128	105	105
1	35	12	38	14	35	24	32	32
2	3	0	0	0	5	2	1	1
3	0	0	0	0	0	0	0	0
total	150	150	148	148	154	154	138	138
mean	0.3	0.1	0.3	0.2	0.3	0.2	0.3	0.3
S.D.	0.2	0.1	0.2	0.2	0.2	0.2	0.2	0.2
percentage change	-63		-40		-33		-0	
p	<0.001		<0.001		<0.001		=0.500	

Table 36.4 includes the initial and final original and mean tooth mobility ratings of those subjects receiving systemic therapy versus placebo supplementation. There appears to be approximately a 63 percent reduction in the mean tooth mobility values ($p<0.001$) in the group which was administered natural vitamin C and bioflavonoids. Those receiving synthetic vitamin C and bioflavonoids showed an improvement of 40 percent in their clinical tooth mobility scores ($p<0.001$). In order, the synthetic vitamin C group followed with approximately 33 percent improvement ($p<0.001$). Finally, the placebo group

showed no change in clinical tooth mobility scores.

Within the limits of this study, the evidence suggests that adding the water soluble bioflavonoids to vitamin C enhances the efficacy of the treatment. There is also some data to suggest that the natural vitamin C may be more efficacious than the synthetic vitamin C with water soluble bioflavonoids.

Parenthetic mention should be made that these relationships have also been studied with regard to gingival inflammation and to periodontal pocket depth and the publications describing the results are listed in the Appendix. All that need be said here is that the findings demonstrated in this report with clinical tooth mobility is very much the same as the observations made with the other two periodontal parameters.

PART

FIVE

DIET

AND

VITAMIN

C

STATE

Man does not live by vitamin C alone!

Emanuel Cheraskin

37. What About the Effect of Dietary Vitamin C upon Vitamin C State?

As one might expect, practically all of the published material with regard to the effect of diet upon vitamin C state deals with ascorbic acid either in the form of foods or by means of supplementation.

It is generally agreed that disease begins far in advance of its clinical expression. In other words, long before there are symptoms and signs of disease, the pathologic process is already operating at the cellular level. Thus, the continuing problem of clinical investigation is to discover criteria and invent methods for the earliest possible recognition of the disease process.

In this connection, it is generally accepted that tolerance testing is a more sensitive index of disease than single determinations and procedures. The basis for this belief and an analysis of tolerance testing is the theme of this report of sixteen presumably healthy dental students. This study was subsequently published as "The Intradermal Ascorbic Acid Test. Part IV. A Study of Tolerance Testing in Sixteen Dental Students" which appeared in the Journal of Dental Medicine (14: #3, 131-155, July 1959).

Specifically, plasma ascorbic acid levels and intradermal decolorization test times were performed simultaneously in sixteen dental students. Immediately following these determinations, one gram of sodium ascorbate was administered intravenously to each of the students. The plasma ascorbic acid and intradermal time values were then redetermined fifteen minutes after the intravenous injection, and again at 24 and 48 hours postinjection. In addition, a history of dietary intake of citrus fruit juices was acquired. A dietary consumption of three or less 6-ounce glasses of citrus juice or its equivalent per week was considered a **poor** citrus intake. A diet containing more than three 6-ounce glasses or its equivalent per week was accepted as a **good** citrus intake.

Figure 37.1 represents the 48-hour tolerance response of the 16 dental students. It can be seen that the mean plasma ascorbic acid level rose from an initial pretolerance value of 0.53 to 1.26 mg. percent 15 minutes postinjection. Clearly, this difference is statistically significant (p<0.001).

Figure 37.1

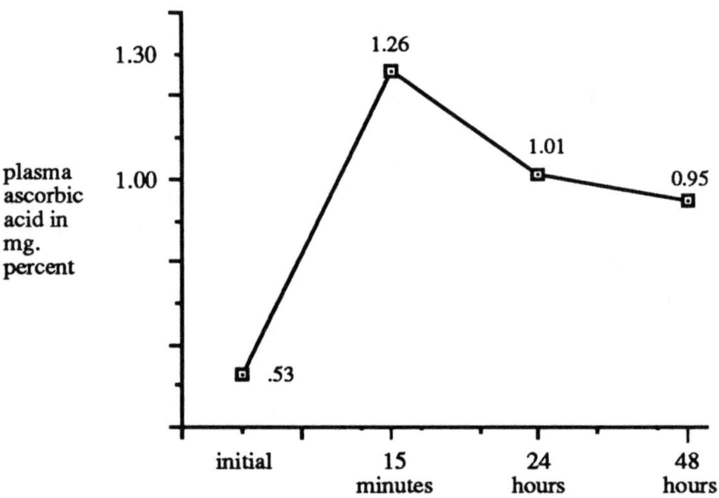

The descent from 1.26 to 1.01 mg. percent was also significant (p<0.005). The ostensible fall from 1.01 to 0.95 mg. percent from 24 to 48 hours was not statistically significant (p>0.500). That the 48-hour level was significantly higher than the initial score is also clear (p<0.005).

Thus, the group response to ascorbic acid loading, as visualized in plasma changes in a group of presumably healthy young people, is a pronounced initial rise 15 minutes after an intravenous injection of 1 gram of ascorbic acid and a slight decrease at 24 hours and no appreciable changes at 48 hours. However, it should be underlined that the 48-hour plasma ascorbic acid concentration remained above the initial pretolerance level.

Figure 37.2 shows the divergent plasma responses of persons with good versus poor citrus intake habits. The tolerance pattern of the good diet group is one of an elevation in plasma ascorbic acid level at 15 minutes and a continued elevated level at both 24 and 48 hours. In contrast, those on a poor citrus diet show a pronounced decrease at 24 and 48 hours. The reduction in plasma level brings the 48-hour concentration to a point not significantly different from the initial baseline.

It is interesting that the plasma levels of both groups tend to be similar at 15 minutes postinjection. At no other point is this likeness in evidence. This is further suggestive that some limit, common to both groups, is being approached.

Figure 37.2

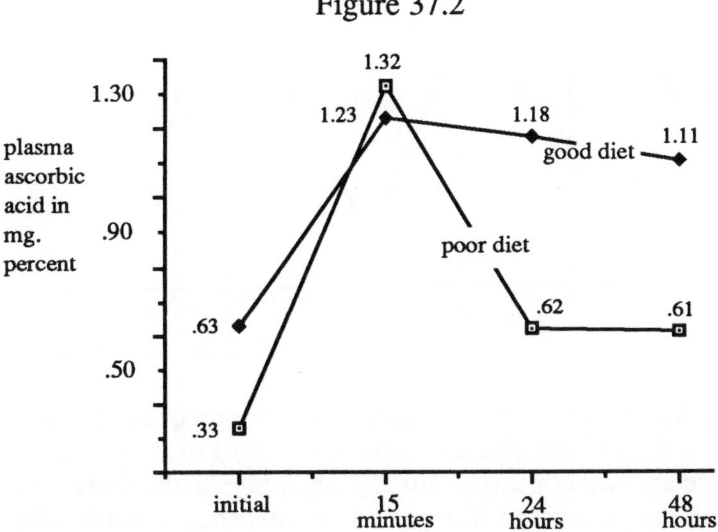

The overall pattern for the intradermal time is also pictorially portrayed (Figure 37.3). This is almost a mirror image of the general plasma ascorbic acid response to the intravenous injection of 1 gram of ascorbic acid. Clearly, there is a statistically significant difference between the initial and 15-minute postinjection scores and between the 15-minute and 24-hour scores. Thus, the general sequence is one of a decline in time at 15 minutes, ascent at 24 hours. The 48-hour scores are essentially not different from the original levels.

Figure 37.4 displays the comparative intradermal tolerance responses of persons on a good versus those on

126

a poor citrus regime. Both groups show a decided drop in intradermal time at 15 minutes postinjection and a significant upswing at 24 hours. Both groups returned to their original scores by 48 hours.

Figure 37.3

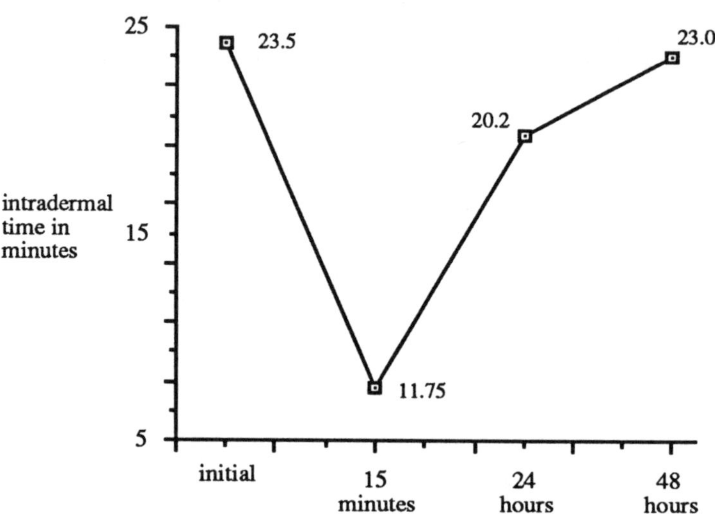

While the plasma ascorbic acid tolerance patterns and those for the intradermal time are overall mirror images, there are two contrasts. Firstly, an analysis of differences from test period to test period reveals that, whereas the group plasma ascorbic acid levels remain raised at 48 hours, the intradermal time has returned to its original level by this time. Secondly, it is of interest that the initial and 48-hour intradermal times exhibited less variability than the plasma ascorbic acid scores at these same test periods.

In summary, the evidence presented from this small study of sixteen healthy subjects is that vitamin C tolerance testing yields more critical information than single test values. Additionally, comparative analysis mildly favors the intradermal tolerance test response as more informative than the plasma ascorbic acid concentration tolerance test.

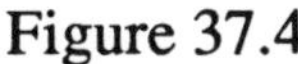

Figure 37.4

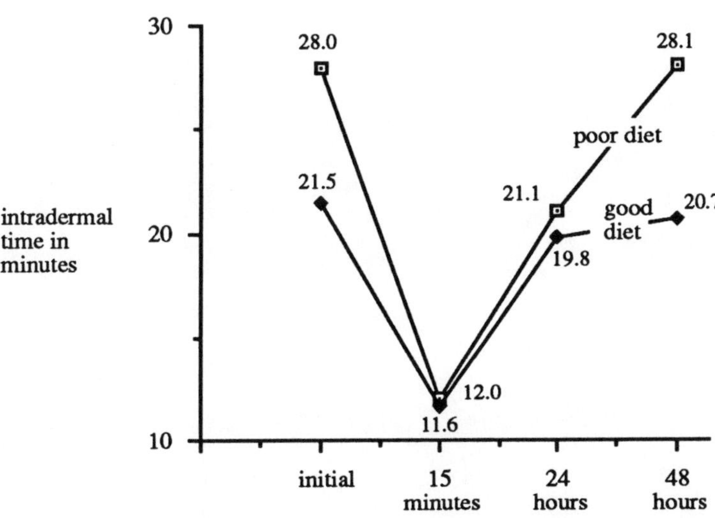

But, most importantly in answer to the question raised in this section, dietary vitamin C significantly alters the vitamin C state!

38. Can Protein Supplementation Influence the Vitamin C State?

Perhaps the most striking impression received from a review of the literature is that hardly any experiment undertaken with any pair of nutrients has failed to show a significant interaction in terms of some nutritional or biochemical criterion.

This should not be surprising since each step in the chain of reactions through which a nutrient passes as it follows an appropriate metabolic pathway is mediated by at least one enzyme system. The functioning of every enzyme system calls for the combined action of an apoenzyme (made up for the most part of amino acids) and a coenzyme (which usually includes a vitamin and/or a mineral element).

For these reasons and others, we thought it wise to examine the possible effect of vitamin C state by means of dietary protein. This was eventually accomplished in an experiment which was reported as "A Lingual Vitamin C Test: XVIII. Effect of Protein Upon Vitamin C State" which appeared in the Alabama Journal of Medical Sciences (7: #3, 288-290, July 1970).

Actually, 80 presumably healthy third-year dental students shared in this experiment. All of the participants were subjected to the lingual vitamin C test on Monday and Friday of a week approximately two-hours after breakfast. Group 1 consisted of 44 subjects. One-half received a 40-gram per day amino acid supplement; the remaining half was given a placebo (methylcellulose) supplement indistinguishable from the protein product. Additionally, in another group, consisting of 36 subjects, 19 of the group were administered a 40-gram per day tripe flour supplement; the remaining 17 were provided an indistinguishable placebo (methylcellulose) supplement.

Table 38.1 summarizes in tabular fashion the vitamin C state as measured by the lingual time for the entire sample and for subsets based upon vitamin C state as judged by the tongue test.

Table 38.1

sample	sample size	lingual time initial mean	final mean	differ-ence	t	p
placebo	22	28	31	+3	2.033	>0.050
amino acid	22	32	26	-6	2.225	<0.050**
placebo						
LT* 14-22	11	19	25	+6	2.953	<0.025**
LT* 25-60	11	37	38	+1	0.314	>0.500
amino acid						
LT* 19-28	11	23	21	-2	2.252	<0.050**
LT* 29-55	11	40	32	-8	1.792	>0.100

* initial lingual times
** statistically significant

The record clearly shows that there is a statistically significant reduction of approximately six seconds in the lingual vitamin C test time in the protein-treated group versus the placebo supplemented subjects. Additionally, there are also significant reductions in the lingual time (4 seconds) with the three-day tripe flour protein versus placebo supplementation (Table 38.2). Hence, within the limits of this simple study, there is absolutely no question but that one can improve vitamin C state (as measured by the lingual time) only with protein supplementation.

Additionally, an attempt was made to ascertain whether the initial vitamin C state dictated in any way the relative improvement in ascorbic acid metabolism. For the amino acid group, the greater (statistically speaking) reduction in lingual time (meaning improvement in vitamin C state) was primarily discovered in those subjects with the shorter lingual time (meaning the better vitamin C state initially). In contrast, the greater improvement in the tripe flour group, however, occurred in those with relatively longer lingual test times (meaning poorer vitamin C state).

Under double-blind control and employment of a placebo group, both the amino acid and tripe flour protein supplements produced a statistically significant improvement in tissue ascorbic acid levels. Specifically, a 15 and 19 percent reduction in lingual time occurred following supplementation for four days with an essential amino acid preparation and for tripe flour protein respectively. As pointed out earlier, for the amino acid group, the greater reduction was primarily in those with the shorter lingual times. The greater improvement in the tripe flour group, however, was in those with relatively longer lingual times.

Thus, under these conditions, it would appear that increases in animal protein consumption are beneficial

Table 38.2

sample	sample size	lingual time initial mean	final mean	differ-ence	t	p
placebo	19	26	27	+1	1.538	>0.100
tripe protein	17	27	23	-4	2.943	<0.010**
placebo						
LT* 15-22	10	20	23	+3	1.689	>0.100
LT* 23-40	9	32	32	0	0.214	>0.500
tripe protein						
LT* 16-26	9	23	20	-3	1.960	>0.050
LT* 27-55	8	33	26	-7	2.469	<0.500**

* initial lingual times
** statistically significant

even in the relatively young and healthy. Nutrient relationship is exhibited by the improvement in ascorbic acid status (decrease in lingual test time) following four days of protein supplementation. Adding 40 grams of protein and placebo daily to the diets of these subjects did not materially change their diets, qualitatively or quantitatively. Thus, the intake of other foodstuffs or nutrients was essentially the same.

Parenthetic mention should be made that the vitamin C changes reported here are similar to those described elsewhere with a reduction in refined-carbohydrate consumption (p. 133).

39. What About Sugar and Vitamin C State?

There is suggestive evidence in the scientific literature that there is, at least in the minds of some investigators, a linear relationship between vitamin C and carbohydrate metabolism. In fact, it has been reported that there is a progressive and significant decrease in the glucose tolerance pattern which parallels successive stages of vitamin C depletion in guinea pigs.

More recently, utilizing variations of the glucose tolerance test and the two-hour postprandial blood glucose, there is the suggestion that a correlation (but a parabolic one rather than a linear one) prevails. In other words, relatively low vitamin C levels may be correlated with either relative hypo-or hyperglycemia.

We looked into this problem and reported our findings in a paper entitled "Effect of Low-Refined-Carbohydrate Diet upon Vitamin C State" in the International Journal for Vitamin Research (40: #1, 77-80, 1970).

Table 39.1

sample	sample size	lingual time initial mean	final mean	difference	t	p
entire	40	24	23	-1	0.179	>0.500
LT*11-16	14	13	18	+5	3.035	<0.010**
LT*17-25	13	21	21	0	0.046	>0.500
LT*26-65	13	36	31	-5	5.046	<0.001**

 * initial lingual times (seconds)
** statistically significant

In this particular experiment, 40 allegedly healthy dental students were examined on Monday of a week. This included the lingual vitamin C test. The group was then instructed to reduce, as far as possible, the intake of sucrose and other processed starches (including baked goods, ready-to-eat breakfast cereals, breads). The lingual time was then remeasured on Friday of the same week with no knowledge of the earlier scores.

Table 39.1 summarizes the important findings. While there were no significant differences for the entire sample, the lingual vitamin C test indicated a decrease of an order of 5 seconds in tissue ascorbic acid levels in those with extremely high concentrations of vitamin C and an increase in tissue vitamin C levels where they were poor (also of a magnitude of 5 seconds). The subjects with a relatively physiologic vitamin C level did not change following carbohydrate restriction.

Hence, the evidence seems to suggest that the elimination of a high refined carbohydrate diet seems to exert a homeostatic effect upon vitamin C, meaning that the scores settled into a more narrow and balanced range.

PART

SIX

VITAMIN

C

AND

METABOLISM

Avoid membership in a body of persons pledged to only one side of anything.

Henry S. Haskins

40. Is there any Possible Relationship Between Serum Cholesterol and Vitamin C State?

As one might expect with the burgeoning interest in the possible causes for heart disease, many different major foodstuffs (and especially fats) as well as a number of vitamins and minerals have been looked at with the hope that they may exert a hypocholesterolemic effect.

We examined this problem and reported out a publication entitled "A Lingual Vitamin C Test: VII. Relationship of Nonfasting Serum Cholesterol and Vitamin C State" which was published in the International Journal for Vitamin Research (38: #3/4, 415-420, 1968).

Figure 40.1

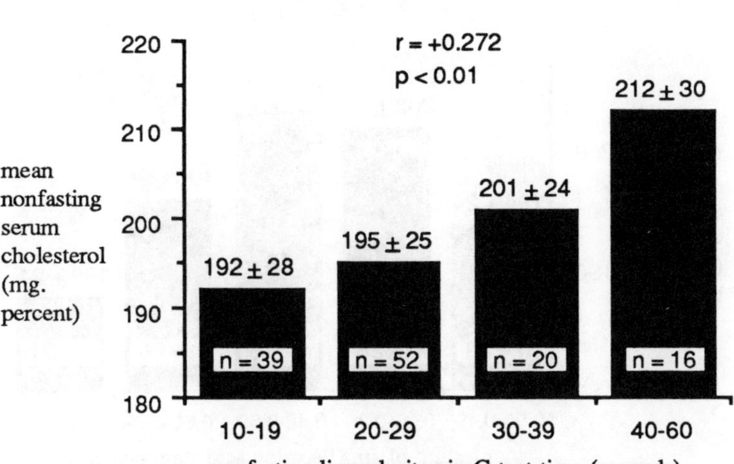

One hundred and twenty seven presumably healthy junior dental students participated in this study. At approximately 10:00 A.M., three hours following breakfast, the serum cholesterol concentration was measured along with the plasma ascorbic acid level and the lingual vitamin C state.

Figure 40.1 outlines on the abscissa the nonfasting lingual vitamin C test scores expressed in seconds. Shown

138

on the ordinate are the mean nonfasting serum cholesterol values.

It will be noted that, on a mean basis, those characterized by the best vitamin C state as judged by the lowest lingual scores (10 to 19 seconds) show the lowest serum cholesterol concentration (192 ± 28 mg. percent). Conversely, the sixteen subjects with the longest vitamin C scores (suggesting the poorest state) show the highest serum cholesterol values (212 ± 30 mg. percent). Finally, those occupying intermediate positions in terms of vitamin C state assumed intermediate positions in terms of serum cholesterol. In short, it will be noted that, on a mean basis, the average serum cholesterol rises as the lingual

Figure 40.2

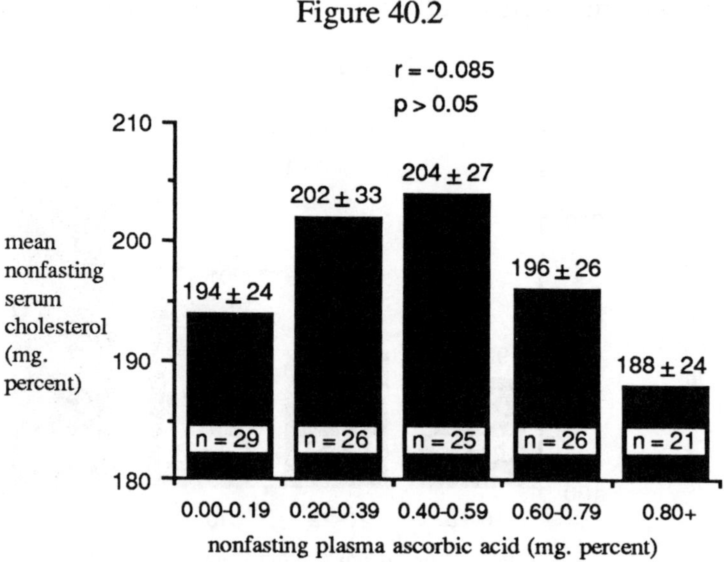

vitamin C test scores increase. The statistical significance is underscored by a correlation coefficient of +0.272 and a p<0.01. Thus, the higher (meaning the poorer) serum cholesterol, the higher (meaning the poorer) lingual vitamin C test scores.

Figure 40.2 describes the nonfasting plasma ascorbic acid levels on the horizontal axis and the mean nonfasting serum cholesterol values on the y-axis. The fact that there is no statistically significant relationship is underscored by r = -0.085 and a p>0.05. Hence, there does not necessarily seem to be a significant relationship between serum cholesterol and dietary vitamin C since vitamin C plasma level principally measures what one ingests.

In other words, to the extent that one can draw conclusions from this report, vitamin C **state** seems to correlate with blood cholesterol level; however, vitamin C intake may not necessarily show this same relationship.

41. Is There any Correlation Between Vitamin C Levels Under Tolerance Conditions in Smokers versus Non-smokers?

The usual statement that appears in the literature is that every cigarette smoked burns up approximately 25 mg. of vitamin C. Beyond that, there has been very little of a quantitative nature in the general literature.

For that and other reasons, we looked at the differences in blood and skin levels in smokers and nonsmokers. We published our results in a paper "The Intradermal Ascorbic Acid Test: Part IV. A Study of Tolerance Testing in Sixteen Dental Students" which appeared in the Journal of Dental Medicine (14: #3, 131-155, July 1959).

Plasma ascorbic acid levels as well as intradermal times were performed in 16 supposedly healthy dental

Figure 41.1

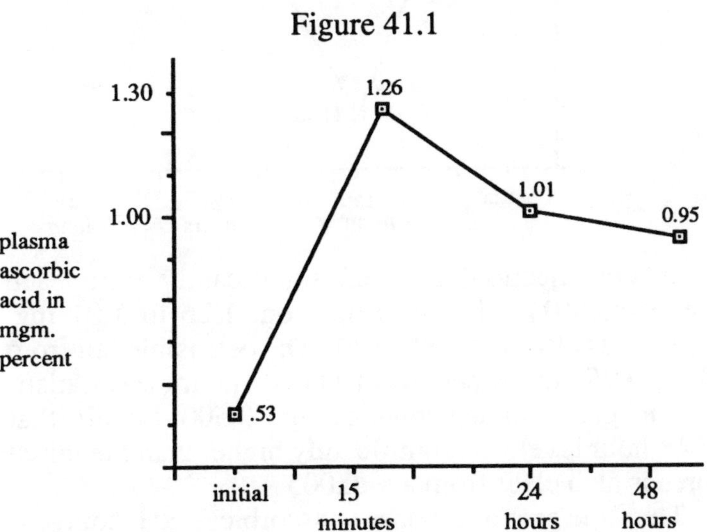

students. Immediately following these determinations, one gram of vitamin C was administered intravenously to each of the students. The plasma ascorbic acid levels were then redetermined at 15 minutes after the intravenous injection and again at 24 and 48 hours postinjection. In addition, a history of smoking habits was taken. This provided an opportunity of studying the different vitamin C responses to an intravenous load in smokers versus nonsmokers.

Figure 41.1 represents the 48-hour tolerance response of the sixteen dental students. It can be seen that the mean plasma ascorbic acid level rose from an initial pretolerance value of 0.53 to 1.26 mg. percent 15 minutes postinjection. Additionally, these two groups (preinjection

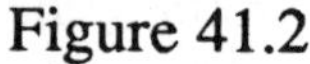

Figure 41.2

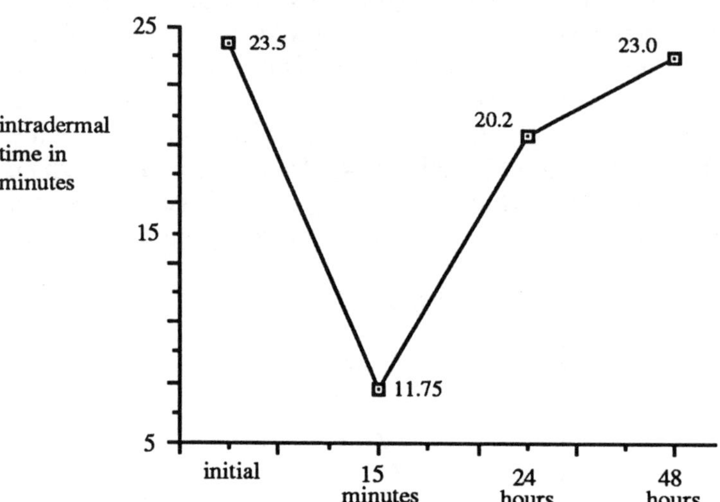

versus postinjection) differed significantly from each other (p<0.001). The descent from 1.26 to 1.01 mg. percent was also real (p<0.005). The ostensible fall from 1.01 to 0.95 mg. percent from 24 to 48 hours was statistically insignificant as shown by a p>0.500. Finally, that the 48-hour level was significantly higher than the initial scores is also clear from a p<0.005.

Thus, the group response to ascorbic acid loading, as visualized in plasma changes in the group of presumably healthy young people, is a pronounced initial rise 15 minutes after an intravenous injection of 1 gram of ascorbic acid, a slight decrease at 24 hours and no appreciable change at 48 hours. However, the 48-hour plasma ascorbic acid concentration remains above the initial pretolerance level.

The intradermal tolerance data is also shown (Figure 41.2). It should be underscored that as intradermal time becomes lower, ascorbic acid levels in the skin increase. Thus, Figure 41.2 represents the average intradermal responses of the sixteen dental students. There is almost a mirror image of the general plasma ascorbic acid response to the intravenous injection of one gram of ascorbic acid.

Figure 41.3 describes the tolerance patterns for the smokers (shown by the dark squares) versus the nonsmokers (depicted by the open, that is, white squares).

Figure 41.3

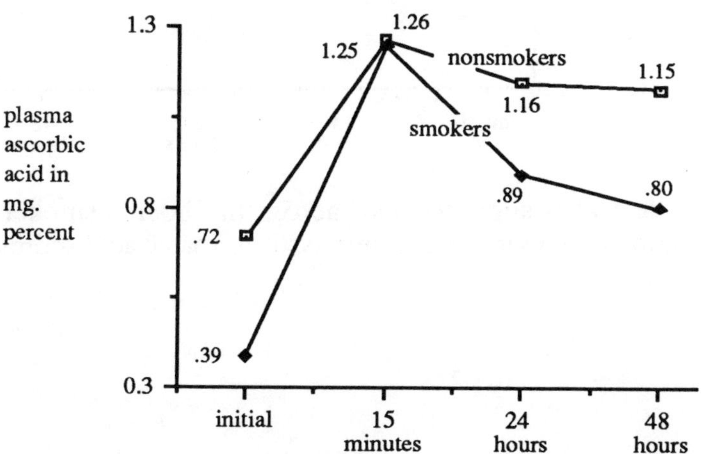

The comparative responses of smokers and nonsmokers is pictorially portrayed. The nonsmoker group plasma level rose at 15 minutes postinjection and remained elevated at 24 and 48 hours. In contrast, the smokers demonstrated a sharp 15-minute postinjection rise but a decline at 24 hours which remained relatively unchanged at 48 hours. Notwithstanding, the 48-hour level of the smoker was still found to be above the baseline determinations.

Finally, Figure 41.4 outlines the different patterns in smokers and nonsmokers as measured by the intradermal ascorbic acid test.

In short, there is no question but that the ascorbic acid

test is significantly different in smokers and nonsmokers.

Figure 41.4

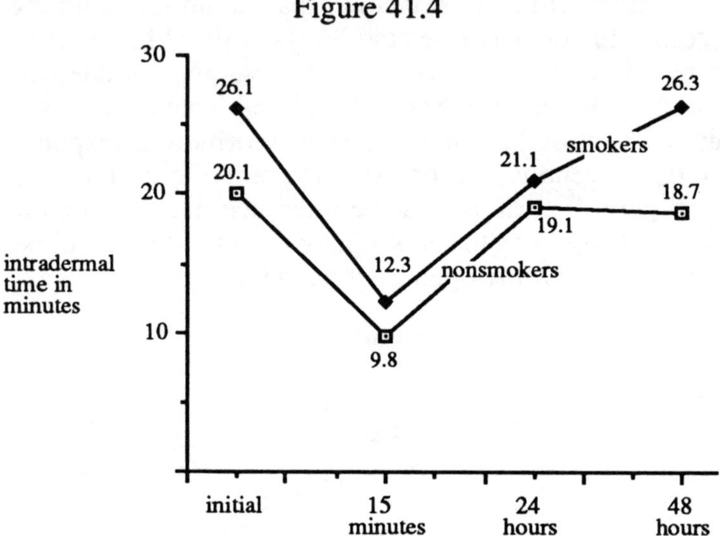

The test also suggests that, across the board, smokers demonstrate poorer blood and tissue ascorbic acid scores.

42. What if Any is the Relationship between Carbohydrate Metabolism and Vitamin C State?

Over almost half a century there has been evidence accumulating from both lower animal and human studies that there is a significant relationship between vitamin C and carbohydrate metabolism. The general consensus has been that a progressive and significant decrease in glucose tolerance (meaning elevated blood glucose) parallels the successive stages of vitamin C depletion in guinea pigs.

The purpose of this report is to investigate whether, in fact, in the human organism, a significant parallelism does indeed exist between the cortisone glucose tolerance test and plasma ascorbic acid concentration.

These results have been published in a paper entitled "Ascorbic Acid and Carbohydrate Metabolism. I. The Cortisone Glucose Tolerance Test" which appeared in the Journal of the American Geriatrics Society (13: #10, 924-934, October 1965).

One hundred sixty-nine presumably healthy persons, drawn at random, participated in this experiment. Most of the subjects were in the third age decade and the sample was predominately female. Carbohydrate metabolism was studied in each person by means of the cortisone glucose tolerance test which, at that time, was considered to be the most sophisticated measure of carbohydrate metabolism.

As an aside, from a search of the literature, there seems to be no argument that age parallels a decrease in glucose tolerance. The question to be resolved is whether the pattern is part of the physiologic aging process or whether it signifies pathosis.

Most authorities do not regard the correlation as representing a grossly pathologic state. The justification for this point of view is based largely on comparatively large numbers of elderly persons, not grossly ill, who show a decrease in glucose tolerance. However, there are others who contend that abnormal glucose tolerance at any age is pathologic. These authorities argue that the common occurrence of a decrease in glucose tolerance in the aging population simply reflects the presence of a common disturbance in carbohydrate metabolism.

Figure 42.1 describes the glucose tolerance pattern for the 89 persons under the age of 36 years (pictured by the open squares) versus the pattern for the 80 subjects 36+

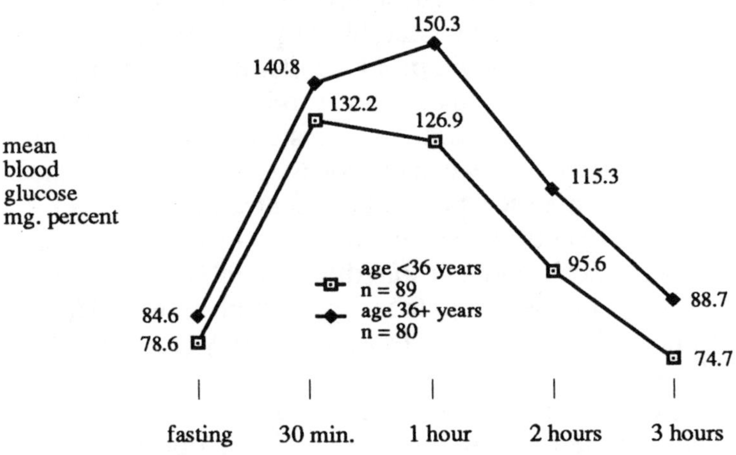

Figure 42.1

cortisone glucose tolerance

years of age (pictured by the dark rectangles). On a mean basis, there is absolutely no question but that, with advancing age, blood glucose levels at almost all temporal points are higher. The statistical significance of this

Table 42.1

significant differences of the means and the variances: age <36 years versus age 36+ years

cortisone glucose tolerance test	age <36 years (n = 89)		age 36+ years (n = 80)		significant difference of the means	significant difference of the variances
	mean	S.D.	mean	S.D.		
fasting	78.6	12.6	84.6	16.2	<0.0100*	<0.0250*
30 min	132.2	32.3	140.8	37.3	>0.0500	<0.0100*
1 hr	126.9	37.0	150.3	48.7	<0.0010*	<0.0100*
2 hrs	95.6	29.0	115.3	44.9	<0.0010*	<0.0005*
3 hrs	74.7	26.6	88.7	40.1	<0.0100*	<0.0005*

* statistically significant.

illustration is underscored in Table 42.1. One notes a statistically significant difference of the means at every temporal point except 30 minutes. There is also a significant difference of the variances at all temporal points.

Figure 42.2 outlines the cortisone glucose patterns on the basis of plasma ascorbic acid (PAA) concentration.

Figure 42.2

cortisone glucose tolerance

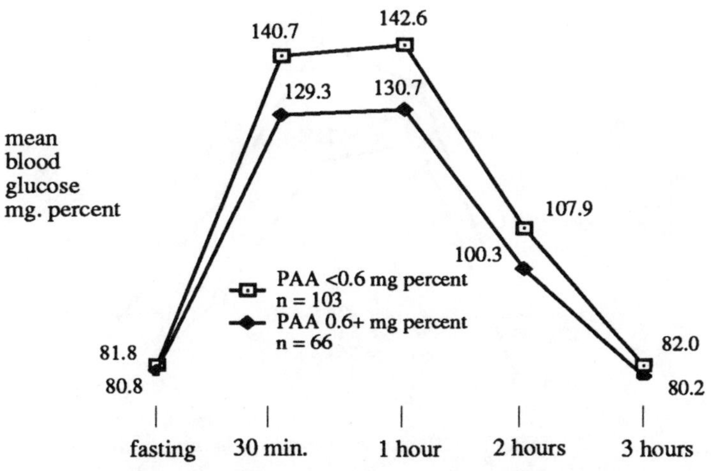

Thus, we see the 103 subjects with a relatively poorer vitamin C level (<0.6 mg. percent) versus 66 subjects with a relatively good plasma C concentration (0.6+ mg.

Table 42.2

significant differences of the means and the variances:
plasma ascorbic acid
level <0.6 mg. percent versus 0.6+ mg. percent

cortisone glucose tolerance test	P.A.A. <0.6 mg/cent (n = 103)		P.A.A. 0.6+ mg/cent (n = 66)		significant difference of the means	significant difference of the variances
	mean	S.D.	mean	S.D.		
fasting	81.8	15.3	80.8	13.7	>0.5000	>0.1000
30 min	140.7	36.0	129.3	26.7	<0.0500*	<0.0050*
1 hr	142.6	49.4	130.7	34.5	>0.0500	<0.0010*
2 hrs	107.9	43.7	100.3	28.4	>0.2000	<0.0005*
3 hrs	82.0	39.2	80.2	25.2	>0.5000	<0.0005*

* statistically significant.

percent). In general, the mean values seem to be slightly higher in those with the poorer plasma ascorbic acid levels. However, an examination of Table 42.2 indicates that, on a mean basis, there are relatively few changes except at 30 minutes. On the other hand, there is

Figure 42.3

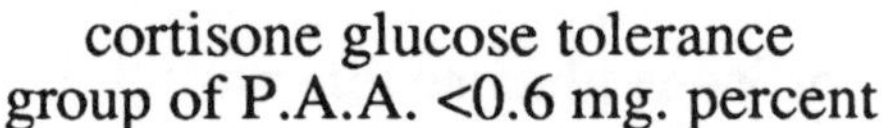

cortisone glucose tolerance
group of P.A.A. <0.6 mg. percent

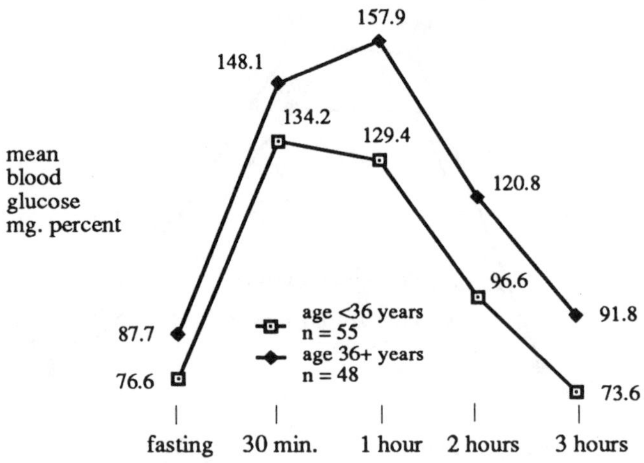

considerable difference in variance at almost every temporal point.

However, it should be emphasized that these findings have been drawn with no consideration to the age factor.

Table 42.3

significant differences of the means and variances: plasma
ascorbic acid level
<0.6 mg. percent; age <36 years versus age 36+ years

cortisone glucose tolerance test	age <36 years (n = 55)		age 36+ years (n - 48)		significant difference of the means	significant difference of the variances
	mean	S.D.	mean	S.D.		
fasting	76.6	12.8	87.7	16.0	<0.0050*	>0.0500
30 min	134.2	27.4	148.1	42.9	>0.0500	<0.0010*
1 hr	129.4	40.0	157.9	54.9	<0.0050*	<0.0250*
2 hrs	96.6	32.2	120.8	51.4	<0.0100*	<0.0005*
3 hrs	73.6	29.6	91.8	46.2	<0.0250*	<0.0010*

* statistically significant.

In order to hone in on the age factor in terms of vitamin C, Figure 42.3 shows the 55 subjects under the age of 36 versus the 48 36+ years of age in those individuals characterized by a relatively low (poorer) vitamin C concentration (<0.6 mg. percent). Here the findings are more sharply defined. At every temporal point, at least on a mean basis, the older subjects seemed to have higher blood glucose scores. This is supported in Table 42.3 where one finds statistically significant differences of the means at almost every temporal point along

Figure 42.4

cortisone glucose tolerance
group of PAA >0.6 mg. percent

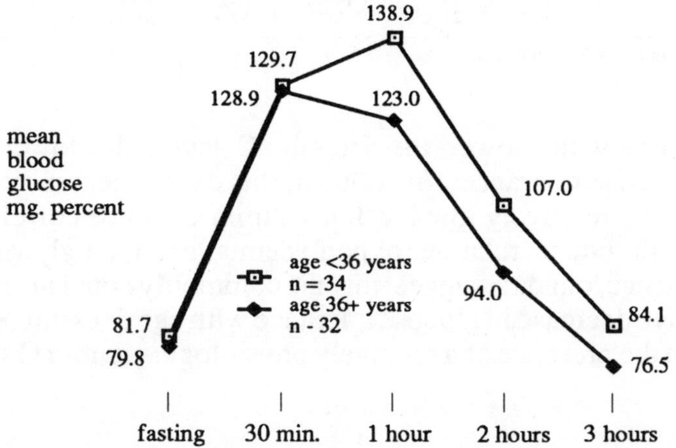

with considerable evidence of a difference in variance.

Finally, to confirm that it is the combination of age and poor vitamin C state that discriminates the glucose tolerance pattern, one should turn to Figure 42.4. Here one finds (confirmed by Table 42.4), no significant differences of the means at any of the temporal points and only isolated instances of a difference in variance.

This study, therefore, supports the published data by showing a significant parallelism between vitamin C metabolism (as measured by the plasma ascorbic acid level) and carbohydrate metabolism (as judged by the cortisone glucose tolerance test). However, the observations reported here are at variance with reported literature in one respect. Other investigators have shown a linear relationship between vitamin C and carbohydrate metabolism,

Table 42.4

significant differences of the means and variances:
plasma ascorbic acid level
>0.6 mg. percent; age <36 years versus age 36+ years

cortisone glucose tolerance test	age <36 years (n = 103)		age 36+ years (n = 66)		significant difference of the means	significant difference of the variances
	mean	S.D.	mean	S.D.		
fasting	81.7	11.9	79.8	15.5	>0.5000	>0.0500
30 min	128.9	29.9	129.7	23.4	>0.0500	>0.0050
1 hr	123.0	31.7	138.9	35.2	>0.0500	>0.2500
2 hrs	94.0	23.3	107.0	31.9	>0.0500	<0.0500*
3 hrs	76.5	21.1	84.1	28.8	>0.2000	<0.0500*

* statistically significant.

namely the lower the vitamin C level, the lower the glucose tolerance. In contrast, this experiment indicates that a relatively low level of vitamin C can be correlated with either relative hypoglycemia or hyperglycemia. Hence, our data suggest that the commonly noted progressive decrease in glucose tolerance with age does not occur in the presence of a relatively physiologic vitamin C state.

43. What Happens to Vitamin C Tissue Levels Following a Three-Day Multivitamin/Trace Mineral versus Placebo Supplement?

There are a number of studies, and some have been cited elsewhere in this monograph, dealing with the effects of vitamin C upon vitamin C state.

We wanted also to look at the larger problem of what happens to vitamin C state when one supplies the usual multivitamin/trace mineral supplement. This has been accomplished and reported under the title "A Lingual Vitamin C Test: XX. Effect of Multivitamin-Mineral Supplementation Upon Vitamin C State" which appeared in the Journal of Oral Medicine (25: #4, 118-120, October/December 1970).

The purpose of this report was to try to answer three questions. First, what is the effect of a three-day multivitamin/mineral versus placebo supplement upon vitamin C state as measured by the lingual vitamin C test?

Forty-two subjects participated in this experiment. One group of 22 received once daily at meal time a placebo capsule. The remaining 20 subjects, at the very same time, were given a multivitamin/mineral supplement. The contents are listed in Table 43.1.

Particular mention should be made that each supplement included 150 mg. ascorbic acid.

The lingual vitamin test, described in a number of other sections in this monograph in great detail, was performed under fasting conditions at the start of the experiment on Monday and again after three days, on Friday of the same week.

It will be noted (Table 43.2) that the mean values and standard deviations were very similar for the entire sample at the very start of the experiment, specifically 25 ± 12 versus 25 ± 10 seconds. Attention is also directed to the fact that, during the experimental period, the rise in lingual test time of 3 seconds in the placebo group is not statistically significant. In contrast, following multivitamin/

trace mineral supplementation, the group mean declined 5 seconds and this is indeed statistically significant (p<0.010). Hence, in answer to the first question, following multivitamin/mineral supplementation, vitamin C state improved as judged by a decrease in lingual vitamin C test time.

Table 43.1

contents of multivitamin-mineral supplement

25,000 units	vitamin A (acetate)
1,000 units	vitamin D (irradiated ergosterol)
10 mg.	thiamin HCL (vitamin B1)
10 mg.	riboflavin (vitamin B2)
100 mg.	niacinamide
5 mg.	pyridoxine HCL (vitamin B6)
20 mg.	D-calcium pantothenate
5 mcg.	vitamin B12 (cobalamin concentrate)
150 mg.	ascorbic acid (vitamin C)
5 I.U.	vitamin E (D-alpha tocopherol acid succinate)
1 mg.	vitamin K (menadione)
300 mg.	kelp powder

average analysis
processed Pacific Coast sea kelp
(macrocystis pyrifera)

moisture	8.00%
crude protein	7.50
crude fiber	7.00
nitrogen-free extract	42.20 (carbohydrates)
fat (ether extract)	0.30
ash	35.00
iodine (I)	0.15-0.20*
calcium (Ca)	1.20
phosphorus (P)	0.30
iron (Fe)	0.10
copper (Cu)	0.0008
magnesium (Mg)	0.76
manganese (Mn)	0.0008
sodium (Na)	3.14
potassium (K)	9.63
chlorine (Cl)	12.21
sulphur (S)	0.93
zinc (Zn)	0.0003

* The iodine content of kelp varies with the season of the year and the location of the kelp beds.

The second question asked, is the effect upon vitamin C state as judged by the lingual vitamin C test, a function of the initial vitamin C state as measured by this particular test procedure? The group of 42 students, in addition to being divided into a placebo and multivitamin group, was further subdivided into two near-equal subgroups based upon initial lingual time. Thus, there were 10 subjects with an initial score of 15 to 20 seconds and 12 individuals with an initial lingual time of 23 to 60 seconds in the placebo group. In the multivitamin/mineral group, 8 individuals showed an initial lingual time of 14 to 21 seconds and 12 with 22 to 50 seconds.

It is clear from Table 43.2 that the subjects in the placebo group with either the short or long lingual times showed no statistically significant change after three days. In contrast, it is noteworthy that the only statistically significant alteration in lingual time in the multivitamin/ mineral group occurred in those who had an initial relatively long lingual time of 22 to 50 seconds meaning a poor

Table 43.2

sample	sample size	initial lingual time mean	final lingual time mean	differ- ence	t	p
placebo	22	25	28	+3	0.718	>0.400
multivitamin- trace mineral	20	25	20	-5	3.129	<0.010**
placebo LT* 15-20	10	17	25	+8	1.652	>0.100
LT* 23-60	12	33	30	-3	0.781	>0.400
multivitamin- trace mineral LT* 14-21	8	18	17	-1	0.248	>0.500
LT* 22-50	12	31	22	-9	3.582	<0.005**

* initial lingual times
** statistically significant

vitamin C state. Specifically, there was a reduction of 9 seconds, on a mean basis in lingual time.

Thus, within the limits of these observations, those with the poorer vitamin C state (as judged by the longer lingual time) showed an improvement when supplied with a multivitamin/mineral supplement for three days.

Finally, what is the possible significance of these results? We had earlier shown in other questions that the administration of 100 mg. of ascorbic acid thrice daily for three weeks yielded a reduction in lingual time from 26 to 16 seconds. A comparison of that earlier release and this one is interesting for two reasons. First, the initial lingual test time scores were very similar in the two studies. Second, the change in lingual time (suggesting improvement in vitamin C state) is greater in the earlier study. This may be due either to the larger vitamin C dosage at that time (300 versus 150 mg. per day) and/or the longer period of administration (three weeks versus three days).

In short, the evidence suggests clearly that, within a very brief period of time, and utilizing a standard multi-vitamin/mineral supplement, it is possible to significantly change vitamin C tissue state.

PART

SEVEN

VITAMIN

C

AS

A

PREDICTIVE

INSTRUMENT

Your only insurance against tomorrow is what you do today!

Sir William Osler

44. Can One Utilize Vitamin C Tissue State as a Predictor of Gingival Response to the Cleaning and Polishing of the Teeth?

There is no question but that seemingly similar subjects treated seemingly similarly by the same practitioner for what seems to be the same conditions so often respond differently. On the one hand, some improve; others remain unchanged; some even worsen.

To study this variability in response, we looked at 25 presumably healthy subjects who were studied by means of the lingual vitamin C test. Additionally, the gingiva surrounding the 6 anterior teeth were graded on a four-point scale. The scores were summed and a mean expressed to two decimals.

Gingival state was examined initially, oral prophylaxis was performed in one-half of the mouth, the gingival state was reexamined three weeks later by the same examiner utilizing the same scoring system with no knowledge of the initial scores or the fact that the vitamin C state was ascertained in the subjects. This material was collected in a paper entitled "A Lingual Vitamin C Test: XV. A Predictor of Gingival Response to Oral Prophylaxis" which appeared in The International Journal for Vitamin Research (39: #1, 86-90, 1969).

The results are summarized in the accompanying chart (Table 44.1). It will be noted that 20 of the subjects showed lingual test time scores <35 seconds and 5 were 35+ seconds. Four points deserve special mention. It is interesting that the initial mean gingival score for those with the better, the lower lingual scores (<35 seconds) is lower (0.90 versus 1.37). Secondly, the table shows that three weeks after prophylaxis, the mean gingival score is lower and therefore better (0.58 versus 1.22) in those with the better vitamin C state. Third, it is clear that the gingival state improvement is greater (36 versus 11 percent) in the group with the better vitamin C state. This same chart summarizes similar analyses utilizing progressively more restricted lingual vitamin C test ranges (e.g. <30 versus 30+ seconds, <25 versus 25+ seconds, etc.).

The findings show a clearcut pattern. In all instances, the subjects with the better vitamin C state show the better

Table 44.1

changes in gingival state with oral prophylaxis on the basis of lingual vitamin C test scores

lingual vitamin C test groups (seconds)	sample size	gingival scores mean and S.D.		percentage difference	t	p
		initial	final			
<35	20	0.90	0.58	-36	7.687	<0.001*
35+	5	1.37	1.22	-11	1.307	>0.200
<30	16	0.85	0.55	-35	6.351	<0.001*
30+	9	1.25	1.00	-20	3.298	<0.025*
<25	12	0.83	0.49	-41	5.449	<0.001*
25+	13	1.15	0.91	-21	4.582	<0.001*
<20	7	0.76	0.42	-45	6.138	<0.001*
20+	18	1.08	0.82	-24	5.070	<0.001*

* statistically significant difference

(lower) initial gingival scores. Secondly, in all instances, following prophylaxis, those with the better vitamin C state demonstrate the better (the lower) gingival scores. Finally, the individuals with the best final gingival grades are those with the lowest (best) lingual vitamin C test scores.

45.   Are There Other Evidences of the Use of Vitamin C as a Predictor of Oral Response to Local Therapy?

Because of the fascination of this concept and in view of the fact that so little work has been done in this area, we wanted to describe another example of the predictability of vitamin C state. This was originally reported as "A Lingual Vitamin C Test: XVI. A Predictor of Sulcus Depth Response to Oral Prophylaxis" which appeared in the International Journal for Vitamin Research (39: #1, 91-94, 1969).

The participants were those earlier described in Question 44 (pages 157-158).

As earlier mentioned, at the initial visit, the lingual vitamin C scores were determined. Sulcus depth was graded to the nearest millimeter in the six anterior teeth on one side of the mouth. The individual scores were summed and expressed as a mean to two decimals. The findings are summarized in Table 45.1.

Table 45.1

lingual vitamin C test groups (seconds)	sample size	sulcus depth scores mean		percentage difference	t	p
		initial	final			
<35	20	1.71	1.56	- 9	3.567	<0.005*
35+	5	2.16	1.96	- 9	1.633	>0.100
<30	16	1.65	1.55	- 6	2.392	<0.050*
30+	9	2.05	1.78	-13	3.582	<0.010*
<25	12	1.61	1.52	- 5	2.200	0.050*
25+	13	1.96	1.74	-11	3.427	0.005*
<20	7	1.47	1.37	- 7	1.736	>0.100
20+	18	1.92	1.74	- 9	3.543	<0.005*

* statistically significant difference

It will be noted that 20 of the subjects showed lingual test time scores <35 seconds and 5 were 35+ seconds. Four points deserve particular emphasis. It is interesting that the initial mean sulcus depth for those with the better lingual scores (<35 seconds) is lower (1.71 versus 2.16 mm). Secondly, three weeks after prophylaxis, the mean sulcus depth is lower and, therefore, better (1.56 versus 1.96 mm) in those with the better vitamin C state. Thirdly, it is clear that the sulcus depth improvement is approximately the same (9 percent) in the two groups. Finally, a statistically significant improvement (p<0.005) occurred only in the group with the better vitamin C state.

Table 45.1 summarizes similar analyses utilizing progressively more restricted lingual vitamin C test ranges (e.g. <30 versus 30+ seconds, <25 versus 25+ seconds, etc.). The mean findings reported for these groups are essentially the same.

It would appear that a tool, to be predictive, should meet three specifications. First, it should correlate with the parameter in question. Table 45.1 shows that this requirement is satisfied. Specifically, at the initial visit, the groups with the better (shorter) lingual times are indeed those with the shallower sulci. Secondly, the instrument should forecast in advance of therapy any extent of change. Table 45.1 underlines this point; in each set of groups, those with the shorter (better) lingual times show a lower mean sulcus depth following an oral prophylaxis than the poorer vitamin C groups. Finally, a tool gains in its predictive value if, as its range is restricted, its prognostication is enhanced. Table 45.1 shows this to be the case in general. In the final groups, the subjects with the lingual time less than 20 seconds demonstrate the lowest (closest to zero) and, therefore, the best of all categories (1.47 mm).

However, it must be admitted that the predictability for sulcus depth (p. 157-158) is not as great as previously shown for gingival state following oral prophylaxis.

PART

EIGHT

THE

"IDEAL"

VITAMIN

C

STATE

Do not follow where the paths may lead. Go instead where there is no path and leave a trail.

Anonymous

46. Is it Possible to Establish an "Ideal" Daily Vitamin C Intake?

Over the past few years, the adult RDA (Recommended Dietary Allowance) for vitamin C has been set between 45 and 60 mg. per day. The Food and Nutrition Board grants that the RDA is designed to protect against classical scurvy. It makes no claim that this dosage is intended as the **ideal** daily intake for the maintenance of optimal health.

Other investigators, using teleologic, evolutionary, and therapeutic techniques, have concluded that the daily **optimal** vitamin C consumption may well be between 250 and 5000 mg. per day.

We have been studying this problem based on the hypothesis that relatively symptomless and signfree persons are healthier than those with clinical symptoms and signs. Therefore, the intake of such groups might well provide a basis for designating the **ideal** daily vitamin C consumption.

This material has been collected and published in "The 'Ideal' Daily Vitamin C Intake" which appeared in the Journal of the Medical Association of the State of Alabama (46: #12, 39-40, June 1977).

One thousand thirty-eight dentists and their spouses were evaluated in terms of daily reported vitamin C consumption as judged from a food frequency questionnaire. This measuring device evaluated the vitamin C consumed from both food and supplements. At the same time, clinical state was graded by the Cornell Medical Index Health Questionnaire (CMI). The CMI is a self-administered health form consisting of 195 questions. Each question is answered by circling the word "yes" or "no." The questions are phrased so that the affirmative answers indicate pathology. The clinical findings in this particular study represent the total number of affirmative responses (CMI score).

Table 46.1 (line 1) shows the daily vitamin C consumption for the entire group of doctors and their spouses.

In this sample of 1038, the CMI ranged from 0 to 125 with a mean of 15.9. The daily reported vitamin C intake ranged from 15 to 1120 mg. with a mean and standard deviation of 327 ± 188 mg. Parenthetically, this is approximately sevenfold more than the RDA. It should also be mentioned that both the American Medical Association and the American Dental Association have indicated that the type of doctor interested in his own health enough to be studied is probably above average in health. Hence, in the usual context, these values would be viewed as **ideal** when, in fact, they are only normal (average).

Table 46.1

line	sample size	CMI range	CMI mean	vitamin C (mg.) range	vitamin C (mg.) mean & S.D.
1) entire sample	1038	0-125	15.9	15-1120	327±188
2) CMI<50	1015	0-49	14.8	15-1120	328±189
3) CMI<40	986	0-39	14.0	15-1120	331±189
4) CMI<30	912	0-29	12.4	41-1120	335±189
5) CMI<20	740	0-19	9.8	41-1120	339±191
6) CMI<15	581	0-14	7.9	41-1120	349±193
7) CMI<10	372	0-9	5.7	41-1120	352±192
8) CMI<5	113	0-4	2.8	49-1120	376±187
9) CMI<4	73	0-3	2.1	104-736	383±181
10) CMI<3	46	0-2	1.5	108-736	389±185
11) CMI<2	16	0-1	0.6	116-719	390±110
12) CMI 0	6	0	0.0	120-719	410±251

Deleting all subjects with 50+ symptoms and signs leaves a sample size of 1015 (line 2), a mean of 14.8, a vitamin C range of 15–1120 mg. and a mean and standard deviation of 328 ± 189 mg. per day.

Exclusion of all subjects with 40+ symptoms and signs (line 3) nets a sample whose daily vitamin C intake is 331 ± 189.

Proceeding through the twelve lines of this table, the daily vitamin C intake slowly rises as the number of allowable clinical symptoms and signs (CMI score) is reduced. This approach indicates that the healthier the sample, the greater the daily vitamin C intake. Under the conditions of this experiment, approximately 410 mg. of vitamin C may be designated as the **ideal** daily allowance. This is about nine times the RDA.

It should be quickly added that it is recognized that the **ideal** is nonexistent as a theoretic end-point since there is biochemical individuality and because the state of the measurement art leaves much to be desired. Nevertheless, the technique utilized here provides a goal not previously considered.

47.   What is the "Ideal" Intradermal Ascorbic Acid Test Range?

Considerable mention has been made throughout this monograph of the use of the intradermal ascorbic acid test as a measure of tissue, specifically skin, vitamin C concentration. What has not been indicated is what is the physiologic range for this procedure.

In an attempt to establish ideality, 120 pregnant and postpartum Caucasian women were studied in five obstetrical clinics in Birmingham, Alabama. Each patient was queried regarding possible oral symptoms and signs in addition to an oral examination. Intradermal test times were determined at the same visit. This material was collected and culminated as a report "Intradermal Ascorbic Acid Test: Part V. Physiologic Range" which was published in the Journal of Dental Medicine (17: #2, 76-79, April 1962).

It is generally held that, in practically all instances, the accepted range for a particular test is derived from a mean and one or two standard deviations of a **presumably** healthy group of individuals. The presumption is made that, if the patient's score falls within the spread of 68 to 95 percent of the measured population, then the results are physiologically acceptable. The fallacy of this approach is readily demonstrated. Were this technique to be applied to develop the physiologic limits for dental caries, for example, one would necessarily conclude that it is physiologically in order to possess X number (since 95 percent of the population suffer with tooth decay). Obviously, it it now clear that, at least in terms of dental decay, the only acceptable score is zero (a point, in fact, not even a range).

A second approach to establish physiologic spread is to develop values for a particular test in a **symptomless** and **signfree** group of individuals. This is reasonable since the presumption can be made safely that, all other factors being equal, a patient **without** symptoms and signs is probably healthier than one **with** clinical findings.

It should be parenthetically added that, according to conventional standards, the limited literature reports that the physiologic range for the intradermal time is somewhere between four and fifteen minutes.

In an attempt to develop a physiologic intradermal time in a group of relatively symptomless and signfree persons, an analysis of the interadermal time was first calculated for those of the 120 subjects free of a **single** sign. Thus, the 23 persons without periodontal pathosis showed a mean and a standard deviation of 22 ± 10 minutes (Figure 47.1). A similar analysis of the 25 individuals without tooth loss (though some may have had

Figure 47.1

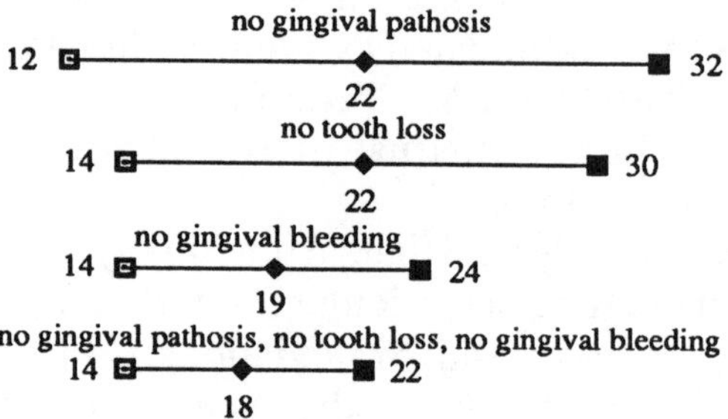

gingival pathosis) yielded 22 ± 8 minutes. It is important to underscore the fact that, though the mean is the same, the range has decreased. A similar plotting of 34 subjects **without** gingival bleeding (though some may have had gingival pathosis and/or tooth loss) showed a mean of 19 minutes and a range of 5 minutes. Finally, the group with 7 persons **without** gingival pathosis, **without** tooth loss, and **without** gingival bleeding shows a mean of 18 minutes with a standard deviation of 4 minutes.

Three points deserve particular mention. Firstly, as one stiffens the specifications for health (the insistence of fewer symptoms and signs) the range continues to shrivel. It might well be that, with even greater stiffening, the range might shrink to zero. Secondly, the lower limits seem to be stationary at about 14 minutes. Thirdly, the upper limit continues to decline from 32 to 30 to 24 and then to 22 minutes.

It would appear, then, that the physiologic intradermal time might well be a point. This still probably cannot be, if for no other reason than there must be an experimental error in performing the test. Incidentally, this has been established at both the inter- and intratechnician level by permitting two technicians to perform the same test at the same time and at different times on the same subject. The error is in the neighborhood of approximately 1 minute.

Thus, the evidence suggests that the **ideal** intradermal time may well be approximately 15 to 20 minutes.

48. Do High and Low Vitamin C Users Differ in Other Dietary Habits?

It is well known that exercisers eat differently from nonexercisers and that cigarette smokers eat differently from nonsmokers.

The question in this report was to analyze the relationship of vitamin C intake to other dietary habits. The results appeared in a paper entitled "The Eating Habits of High and Low Vitamin C Users" in the Journal of Orthomolecular Psychiatry (5: #2, 84-88, 1976).

Table 48.1
the vitamin C profile
(food frequency questionnaire)

factor	<100mg vitamin C per day	400+mg vitamin C per day	percentage change	t	p
(1) vitamin E (units)	19	150	798	35.081	<0.001*
(2) vitamin B_6 (mg)	1.8	7.1	292	34.227	<0.001*
(3) pantothenic acid (mg)	7.5	25.8	243	33.706	<0.001*
(4) vitamin B_3 (mg)	16	137	775	31.288	<0.001*
(5) vitamin B_1 (mg)	1.1	10.3	799	29.847	<0.001*
(6) potassium (mg)	396	3557	798	27.512	<0.001*
(7) vitamin B_2 (mg)	2.1	11.4	45	26.078	<0.001*
(8) vitamin B_{12} (mcg)	4.9	21.8	341	21.105	<0.001*
(9) iodine (mg)	0.38	0.90	135	16.302	<0.001*
(10) iron (mg)	13.5	51.9	284	14.940	<0.001*
(11) isoleucine (mg)	4078	6457	58	11.939	<0.001*
(12) magnesium (mg)	195	384	97	11.565	<0.001*
(13) vitamin A (units)	9391	29628	215	10.505	<0.001*
(14) phosphorus (mg)	1073	1860	73	9.799	<0.001*
(15) methionine (mg)	1624	2391	47	6.622	<0.001*
(16) lysine (mg)	5033	7483	49	6.283	<0.001*
(17) valine (mg)	4138	5929	43	6.174	<0.001*
(18) leucine (mg)	5731	8027	41	6.109	<0.001*
(19) total protein (gm)	84	108	29	6.010	<0.001*
(20) phenylalanine (mg)	3173	4491	42	5.823	<0.001*
(21) threonine (mg)	2914	4083	40	5.565	<0.001*
(22) tryptophane (mg)	898	1235	26	5.231	<0.001*
(23) polyunsaturated fatty acids (mg)	10.4	15.3	47	4.462	<0.001*
(24) percentage polyunsaturated to saturated fat	11.6	17.4	50	4.383	<0.001*
(25) total sodium (mg)	2423	2896	20	3.411	<0.001*
(26) ratio Ca/P	0.61	0.74	21	3.023	<0.005*
(27) total carbohydrate (gm)	154	192	24	2.738	<0.010*
(28) calcium (mg)	939	1375	47	2.635	<0.010*
(29) percentage of calories from refined carbohydrates	29	19	34	2.603	<0.010*

* statistically significant difference of the means

Approximately 700 members of the health professions shared in a multiphasic health examination extending over a period of about seven years. Each year each participant completed the Oral Health Index (OHI) Questionnaire. Additionally, the subjects completed, at each annual examination, a dietary survey. The dietary record, a food frequency questionnaire, was submitted to a computer center which provided a readout showing the daily intake of the major foodstuffs and most of the essential nutrients (vitamins, minerals, amino acids, fatty acids).

With this information it was possible to analyze the overall diet in terms of an assessment of daily vitamin C consumption as shown in the chart (Table 48.1).

The table summarizes the relationship between daily vitamin C consumption and the daily intake of all of the other nutrients as judged by the food frequency questionnaire. The chart also lists the vitamin C and other nutrients in decreasing order of statistical significance as judged by t values and probabilities.

It is abundantly clear that the dietary intake of the nutrients was substantially different in low vitamin C consumers compared with high vitamin C eaters.

For example, it is noteworthy that individuals consuming <100 mg. of vitamin C per day take about 19 I.U. of vitamin E. In contrast, those consuming 400+ mg. of vitamin C per day consume about 150 I.U. of vitamin E— namely, an eightfold difference.

It was found, as shown in the illustration, that, in most instances, those consuming relatively large amounts of vitamin C also consume significantly more of most of the vitamins, minerals, and amino acids. The most notable exception was the fact that the percentage of calories derived from refined carbohydrate foodstuffs was significantly lower in the high vitamin C users.

This experiment raises all kinds of interesting questions with regard to the interplay of nutrients which obviously have not been addressed in this particular experiment. What, in substance, the study does allow us to conclude is that many of the experiments performed in this area must be viewed in the light of the relationship of vitamin C to the consumption of other nutrients.

49. What do we Know About Human Vitamin C Requirements?

There is no denying the heated debate generated by Professor Linus Pauling with the appearance of his paper on orthomolecular psychiatry followed by his book, **Vitamin C and the Common Cold**. One of the controversies stemming from his work is the desired dosage of vitamin C which should be consumed under health versus disease conditions. Interestingly enough, just about the same time, the Food and Nutrition Board of the National Academy of Sciences/National Research Council suggested that the daily vitamin C requirement should be reduced from 60 to 45 mg. per day.

We tried to cast additional light on the daily vitamin C requirements through a study of the reported daily vitamin C intake versus the reported total number of clinical symptoms and signs in presumably healthy groups of doctors and their spouses. We reported this in an article entitled "Human Vitamin C Requirement: Relation of Daily Intake to Incidence of Clinical Signs and Symptoms" which appeared in International Research Communications System (IRCS) (2: #6, 1379, June 1974).

Specifically, each subject completed the Cornell Medical Index Health Questionnaire and the total number of positive responses was noted. Each subject also completed a seven-day dietary survey and the number of milligrams of vitamin C consumed each day was calculated.

The 1071 observations were divided into three groups based on reported daily vitamin C intake. Table 47.1 shows that the 347 subjects consuming less than 100 mg. of vitamin C daily showed a total clinical score of 17.8 ± 12.6. In contrast, the 525 subjects consuming 100 to 199 mg. per day revealed a total clinical score of 15.8 ± 12.6. The difference is statistically significant (t=2.287, p<0.025). The 199 subjects consuming 200+ mg. of vitamin C per day showed a clinical score of 14.6 ± 12.6 which was not statistically significantly different from the group

174

consuming 100 to 199 mg. per day (t=1.128, p>0.200). However, the group consuming the least and the group consuming the greatest amount of vitamin C were indeed very significant (t=2.843, p<0.005).

Figure 49.1

total number of clinical symptoms and signs
(mean and standard deviation)

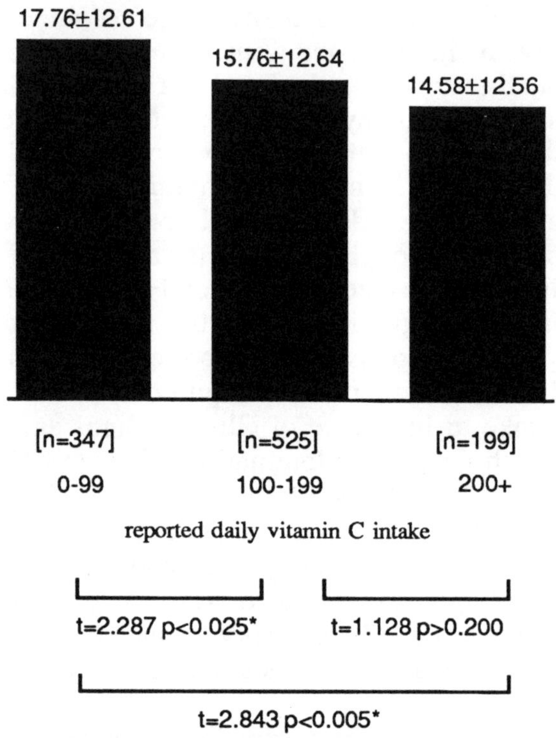

If one grants that the lower the clinical score (the fewer the number of symptoms and signs) the healthier the group, then it is obvious that those consuming 200+ mg. of vitamin C per day represent the healthiest group. This then means that the daily vitamin C intake is approximately four or more fold greater than that recommended by the Food and Nutrition Board of the National Academy of Sciences/National Research Council.

The important point to underline is that the evidence from this simple experiment as well as others suggests that the present RDA, and the one recommended for a number of years, leaves much to be desired in terms of optimal health.

50. What Can We Say About the "Ideal" Lingual Vitamin C Test Score Range?

The generally accepted physiologic range for a particular test is usually derived from the mean and one or two standard deviations of a presumably healthy group of human subjects. The presumption is made that, if the patient's score falls within the spread of 68 to 95 percent of the measured population, his or her results are within the physiologic range.

Frequent reference has been made in this monograph to the measurement of vitamin C in the tongue surface. Nothing has been mentioned up to this point regarding the possible physiologic range. Hence, we made a point of studying this problem which was eventually published in an article entitled "A Lingual Vitamin C Test: XIX. Normal Versus Physiologic Range" which appeared in the Journal of the Ontario Dental Association (47: #10, 239-242, October 1970).

Table 50.1
age distribution

age groups	number of subjects	percentage of subjects
20-24	48	38.7
25-29	59	47.6
30-34	16	12.9
35-39	1	0.8
total	124	100.0
mean		26.1
S.D.		2.8

One hundred twenty-four allegedly healthy male dental students participated in this project. Table 50.1 outlines the age distribution and mean and standard deviation.

Each of the 124 subjects was questioned regarding

178

general health and the presence of oral symptoms. The oral cavity was examined carefully in each individual. Finally, a two-hour postprandial lingual vitamin C time was recorded. This test technique has been described elsewhere in this monograph (p. 21).

Figure 50.1 is an attempt to develop in pictorial fashion the physiologic nonfasting lingual time through a progressive selection of more symptomless and signfree students. The coding for Figure 50.1 is shown in Table 50.2. It will be noted that "a" represents the entire sample of 124 students, "b" indicates the 113 with a negative systemic history, "c" includes the negative systemic history described in "b" along with a negative story of general symptoms and signs in 88 subjects, "d" signifies the 65 individuals with no general symptoms plus no tooth loss. In this way, it is possible to pictorialize the relatively symptomless and signfree individual.

Table 50.2

a = entire sample (n=124)
b = negative systemic history (n=113)
c = negative systemic history plus
    negative general symptoms (n=88)
d = negative general symptoms plus
    no tooth loss (n=65)
e = no tooth loss plus
    negative oral symptoms (n=45)
f = negative oral symptoms plus
    no tooth mobility (n=33)
g = no tooth mobility plus
    no tongue pathosis (n=22)

Utilizing the traditional approach to the establishment of health standards, it must be concluded that the physiologic limits for the lingual test should be 15 to 39 seconds. However, it is noteworthy that, by employing different criteria for health, the mean nonfasting lingual time slowly falls toward approximately 20 seconds. Also, it is of interest that by stiffening the specifications for health (for instance, progressively utilizing subjects with fewer symptoms and signs), the ranges shrivel markedly.

It would be interesting to speculate what the physiologic spread of the lingual time would be if a large sample could be used so that other health criteria might be made even more rigid then described here.

Figure 50.1

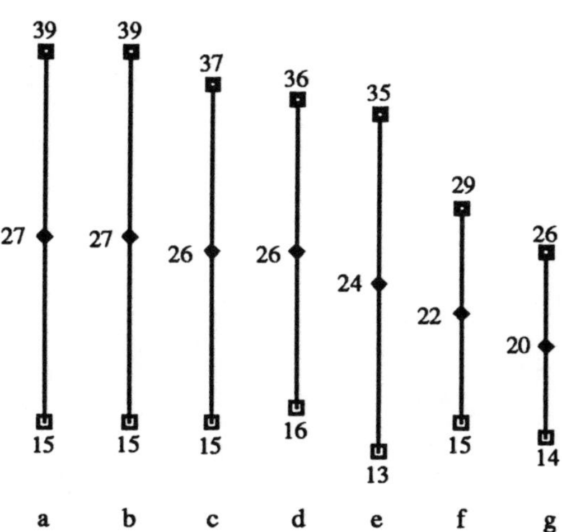

It may well be that the physiologic nonfasting lingual time is indeed a point. This very possibly cannot be since there is always an experimental error in performing a test. An attempt was made to establish this error in Table 50.3 by repeating the lingual vitamin C test fifteen minutes after the initial test.

Table 50.3
lingual test reproducibility

	first reading	second reading
mean	23.4	25.8
standard deviation	10.5	11.5
significance of the difference of the means	P >0.100	
coefficient of correlation	r +0.986	
significance of correlation	P <0.001*	

* statistically significant

Clearly, there is a small error. However, the overall correlation coefficient is very high (r=+0.986) and very significant (p<0.001).

APPENDIX

VITAMIN

C

PUBLICATIONS

In the following pages are listed in chronologic order from 1959 to 1986 all of our published papers dealing with vitamin C.

1. Cheraskin, E., Dunbar, J. B., and Flynn, F. H.
**The Intradermal Ascorbic Acid Test. Part
I. A Review of Animal Studies.**
J. Dent. Med. 12: #4, 174-184, October 1957.

2. Dunbar, J. B., Cheraskin, E., and Flynn, F. H.
**The Intradermal Ascorbic Acid Test. Part
II. A Review of Human Studies.**
J. Dent. Med. 13: #1, 19-40, January 1958.

3. Cheraskin, E., Dunbar, J. B., and Flynn, F. H.
**The Intradermal Ascorbic Acid Test. III.
A Study of Forty-two Dental Students.**
J. Dent. Med. 13: #3, 135-155, July 1958.

4. Karlson, F. A., Jr., Cheraskin, E., and Dunbar, J. B.
**Subclinical Scurvy and Subclinical Tooth
Mobility.**
J. West. Soc. Periodont. 7: #1, 6-28, March 1959.

5. Dunbar, J. B., Cheraskin, E., Flynn, F. H., and
Marley, J. F.
**The Intradermal Ascorbic Acid Test. IV. A
Study of Tolerance Testing in Sixteen Den-
tal Students.**
J. Dent. Med. 14: #3, 131-155, July 1959.

6. Cowan, R. G., Huffstutler, B. B., Cheraskin, E.,
and Dunbar, J. B.
Operation Human Guinea Pig.
J. Appl. Nutr. 12: #3, 98-116, November 1959.

7. Cheraskin, E., Flynn, F. H., Hutto, A. C., Fess,
L. R., Huffstuttler, B. B. and Bockler, C. E.
**The Alabama Study of Maternal Ascorbic
Acid Nutrition. I. General Information.**
Alabama Dent. Rev. 13-29, Spring 1960.

8. Ringsdorf, W. M., Jr. and Cheraskin, E.
**Intradermal Ascorbic Acid Test: Part V.
Physiologic Range.**
J. Dent. Med. 17: #2, 76-79, April 1962.

184

9. Thomas, A. E., Busby, M. C., Jr., Ringsdorf, W.
    M., Jr., and Cheraskin, E.
    Ascorbic Acid and Alveolar Bone Loss.
    Oral Surg., Oral Med., and Oral Path. 15: #5, 555-
    565, May 1962.

10. Ringsdorf, W. M., Jr. and Cheraskin, E.
    **A Rapid and Simple Lingual Ascorbic
    Acid Test.**
    GP 25: #6, 106-108, June 1962.

11. Ringsdorf, W. M., Jr. and Cheraskin, E.
    **A Lingual Vitamin C Test for Periodontic
    Diagnosis.**
    Odont. Revy 14: #1, 23-31, 1963.

12. El-Ashiry, G., Ringsdorf, W. M., Jr., and
    Cheraskin, E.
    **A Lingual Vitamin C Test: Reproducibil-
    ity of Various Test Solutions.**
    Quart. Nat. Dent. Assoc. 22: #1, 16-27, October
    1963.

13. Ringsdorf, W. M., Jr. and Cheraskin, E.
    Simple Lingual Test for Vitamin C Status.
    Dent. Abs. 8: #10, 622-623, October 1963.
    (abstract)

14. Thomas, A. E., Busby, M. C., Jr., Ringsdorf, W.
    M., Jr., and Cheraskin, E.
    Gingival Hue and Orange Juice.
    J. Dent. Med. 18: #4, 171-174, October 1963.

15. Cheraskin, E., Ringsdorf, W. M., Jr., and
    El-Ashiry, G.
    A Lingual Vitamin C Test.
    Int. J. Vit. Res. 34: #1, 31-38, 1964.

16. El-Ashiry, G. M., Ringsdorf, W. M., Jr., and
    Cheraskin, E.
    **Local and Systemic Influences in Perio-
    dontal Disease: II. Effect of Prophylaxis
    and Natural Versus Synthetic Vitamin C
    Upon Gingivitis.**
    J. Periodontol. 35: #3, 250-259, May-June 1964.

17. El-Ashiry, G. M., Ringsdorf, W. M., Jr., and
     Cheraskin, E.
     **Local and Systemic Influences in Perio-
     dontal Disease: IV. Effect of Prophylaxis
     and Natural Versus Synthetic Vitamin C
     Upon Clinical Tooth Mobility.**
     Int. J.Vit. Res. 34: #2, 202-218, 1964.

18. El-Ashiry, G. M., Ringsdorf, W. M., Jr., and
     Cheraskin, E.
     **Local and Systemic Influences in Perio-
     dontal Disease: III. Effect of Prophylaxis
     and Natural Versus Synthetic Vitamin C
     Upon Sulcus Depth.**
     New York J. Dent. 34: #7, 254-262, August-
     September 1964.

19. Cheraskin, E. and Ringsdorf, W. M., Jr.
     **Vitamin C State in a Dental School Patient
     Population.**
     South. Calif. State Dent. Assoc. J. 32: #10, 375-
     378, October 1964.

20. Cheraskin, E. and Ringsdorf, W. M., Jr.
     Vitamins in Health and Disease.
     J. Dent. Med. 19: #4, 147-165, October 1964.

21. Setyaadmadja, A. T. S. H., Cheraskin, E., and
     Ringsdorf, W. M., Jr.
     **Ascorbic Acid and Carbohydrate Metabo-
     lism. I. The Cortisone-Glucose Tolerance
     Test.**
     J. Amer. Geriat. Soc. 13: #10, 924-934, 1965.

22. Setyaadmadja, A. T. S. H., Cheraskin, E., and
     Ringsdorf, W. M., Jr.
     **Ascorbic Acid and Carbohydrate Metabo-
     lism. II. Effect of Supervised Sucrose
     Drinks Upon Two-hour Postprandial Blood
     Glucose in Terms of Vitamin C State.**
     J. Lancet 87: #1, 18-21, January 1967.

23. Collins, C. K., Lewis, A. E., Ringsdorf, W. M., Jr., and Cheraskin, E.
Effect of Ascorbic Acid on Oral Healing in Guinea Pigs.
Int. J. Vit. Res. 37: #4, 492-495, 1967.

24. Cheraskin, E. and Ringsdorf, W. M., Jr.
A Lingual Vitamin C Test: I. Reproducibility.
Int. J.Vit. Res. 38: #1, 114,117, 1968.

25. Cheraskin, E. and Ringsdorf, W. M., Jr.
A Lingual Vitamin C Test: II. Daily Constancy.
Int. J. Vit. Res. 38: #1, 118-119, 1968.

26. Cheraskin, E. and Ringsdorf, W. M., Jr.
A Lingual Vitamin C Test: III. Relationship to Plasma Ascorbic Acid Level.
Int. J. Vit. Res. 38: #1, 120-122, 1968.

27. Cheraskin, E. and Ringsdorf, W. M., Jr.
A Lingual Vitamin C Test: IV. Relationship to Intradermal Time.
Int. J. Vit. Res. 38: #1, 123-126, 1968.

28. Cheraskin, E. and Ringsdorf, W. M., Jr.
A Lingual Vitamin C Test: V. A Study in Dietary Relationships.
Int. J. Vit. Res. 38: #2, 254-256, 1968.

29. Cheraskin, E. and Ringsdorf, W. M., Jr.
A Lingual Vitamin C Test: VI. Effect of Three Week Vitamin C Versus Placebo Supplementation.
Int. J. Vit. Res. 38: #2, 257-259, 1968.

30. Cheraskin, E. and Ringsdorf, W. M., Jr.
A Lingual Vitamin C Test: VII. Relationship of Nonfasting Serum Cholesterol and Vitamin C State.
Int. J. Vit. Res. 38: #3/4, 415-420, 1968.

31. Cheraskin, E. and Ringsdorf, W. M., Jr.
A Lingual Vitamin C Test: VIII. Vitamin C State in a Dental Prepayment Program.
Int. J. Vit. Res. 38: #3/4, 421-423, 1968.

32. Cheraskin, E., Ringsdorf, W. M., Jr., Aspray, D. W., Michael, D., and Preskitt, D.
A Lingual Vitamin C Test: IX. Relationship to Gingival State.
Int. J. Vit. Res. 38: #3/4, 425-432, 1968.

33. Cheraskin, E., Ringsdorf, W. M., Jr., Aspray, D.W., Michael, D., and Preskitt, D.
A Lingual Vitamin C Test: X. Relationship to Tooth Mobility.
Int. J. Vit. Res. 38: #3/4, 433-437, 1968.

34. Cheraskin, E., Ringsdorf, W. M., Jr., Aspray, D. W., and Preskitt, D.
A Lingual Vitamin C Test: XI. Relationship to Gingival Sulcus Depth.
Int. J. Vit. Res. 38: #5, 512-516, 1968.

35. Cheraskin, E., Ringsdorf, W. M., Jr., Aspray, D. W., and Preskitt, D.
A Lingual Vitamin C Test: XII. Relationship to Alveolar Bone Loss.
Int. J. Vit. Res. 38: #5, 517-523, 1968.

36. Cheraskin, E., Ringsdorf, W. M., Jr., Aspray, D. W., and Preskitt, D.
A Lingual Vitamin C Test: XIII. Relationship to Oral Hygiene.
Int. J. Vit. Res. 38: #5, 524-530, 1968.

37. Cheraskin, E. and Ringsdorf, W. M., Jr.
A Lingual Vitamin C Test: XIV. Relationship to Oral Calculus.
Int. J. Vit. Res. 38: #5, 531-537, 1968.

38. Cheraskin, E. and Ringsdorf, W. M., Jr.
A Lingual Vitamin C Test. XV. A Predictor of Gingival Response to Oral Prophylaxis.
Int. J. Vit. Res. 39: #1, 86-90, 1969.

188

39. Cheraskin, E. and Ringsdorf, W. M., Jr.
     **A Lingual Vitamin C Test. XVI. A Pre-
     dictor of Sulcus Depth Response to Oral
     Prophylaxis.**
     Int. J. Vit. Res. 39: #1, 91-94, 1969.

40. Cheraskin, E. and Ringsdorf, W. M., Jr.
     **Biology of the Orthodontic Patient: I.
     Plasma Ascorbic Acid Levels.**
     Angle Orthodont. 39: #2, 137-138, April 1969.

41. Clark, J. W., Cheraskin, E., and Ringsdorf, W. M.,
     Jr.
     An Ecologic Study of Oral Hygiene.
     J. Periodont.-Periodontics 40: #8, 476-480,
     August 1969.

42. Cheraskin, E. and Ringsdorf, W. M., Jr.
     **Biology of the Orthodontic Patient: II.
     Lingual Vitamin C Test Scores.**
     Angle Orthodont. 39: #4, 324-325, October 1969.

43. Cheraskin, E., and Ringsdorf, W. M., Jr.
     **Effect of Regular Versus Sustained Re-
     lease Multivitamin Supplementation upon
     Periodontal Parameters: I. Gingival State.**
     Int. J. Vit. Res. 39: #3, 314-319, 1969.

44. Richards, T. W., Cheraskin, E., and
     Ringsdorf, W. M., Jr.
     **Effect of Sustained-Release Versus Regu-
     lar Multivitamin Supplementation upon
     Vitamin C State.**
     Int. J. Vit. Res. 39: #4, 407-415, 1969.

45. Cheraskin, E., and Ringsdorf, W. M., Jr.
     **Effect of Regular Versus Sustained-
     Release Multivitamin Supplementation
     upon Periodontal Parameters: II. Sulcus
     Depth and Clinical Tooth Mobility.**
     Int. J. Vit. Res. 39: #4, 476-485, 1969.

46. Cheraskin E. and Ringsdorf, W. M., Jr.
Effect of Low-Refined-Carbohydrate Diet Upon Vitamin C State.
Int. J. Vit. Res. 40: #1, 77-80, 1970.

47. Cheraskin, E., and Ringsdorf, W. M., Jr.
A Lingual Vitamin C Test: XVIII. Effect of Protein upon Vitamin C State.
Alabama J. Med. Sci. 7: #3, 288-290, July 1970.

48. Cheraskin, E. and Ringsdorf, W. M., Jr.
A Lingual Vitamin C Test: XIX. Normal Versus Physiologic Range.
J. Ontario Dent. Assoc. 47: #10, 239-242, October 1970.

49. Cheraskin, E. and Ringsdorf, W. M., Jr.
A Lingual Vitamin C Test. XX. Effect of Multivitamin-Mineral Supplementation Upon Vitamin C State.
J. Oral Med. 25: #4, 118-120, October-December 1970.

50. Cheraskin, E. and Ringsdorf, W. M., Jr.
Ecology of Alveolar Bone Loss.
Oral Surg., Oral Med., & Oral Path. 30: #3, 333-350, September 1970.

51. Cheraskin, E. and Ringsdorf, W. M., Jr.
Ecology of Alveolar Bone Loss.
Geriat. Dig. 8: #6, 30, June 1971. (abstract)

52. Cheraskin, E. and Ringsdorf, W. M., Jr.
Biology of the Orthodontic Patient: III. Relationship of Chronologic and Dental Age in Terms of Vitamin C State.
Angle Orthodontist 42: #1, 56-59, January 1972.

53. Cheraskin, E., Ringsdorf, W. M., Jr., Michael, D.W., and Hicks, B. S.
Daily Vitamin C Consumption and Reported Respiratory Findings.
Int. J. Vit. Nutr. Res. 43: #1, 42-55, 1973.

54. Cheraskin, E. and Ringsdorf, W. M., Jr.
**Vitamin C and Chronologic Versus Bone
Age.**
J. Oral Med. 28: #3, 77-80, July-September 1973.

55. Cheraskin, E.
The Name of the Game is the Name.
Proc. San Diego Biomed. Sympos. 1974. 13: 31-
39, 6/8 February 1974.

56. Cheraskin, E., Ringsdorf, W. M., Jr. and Hicks,
B. S.
**Daily Vitamin C Consumption and
Reported Cardiovascular Findings.**
J. Int. Acad. Prev. Med. 1: #1, 31-44, Spring 1974.

57. Cheraskin, E. and Ringsdorf, W. M., Jr.
**Human Vitamin C Requirement: Relation
of Daily Intake to Incidence of Clinical
Signs and Symptoms.**
J. Int. Res. Comm. (IRCS) 2: #6, 1379, June 1974.

58. Cheraskin, E.
The Ecology of Periodontal Disease.
Report Proceed. Workshop on Diet, Nutr. &
Periodont. Dis., Amer. Soc. Prev. Dent., Sun
Valley, Idaho, 7-27, 4-7 August 1974.

59. Cheraskin, E., Ringsdorf, W. M., Jr., and
Medford, F. H.
**Daily Vitamin C Consumption and Fatiga-
bility.**
J. Amer. Geriat. Soc. 24: #3, 136-137, March 1976.

60. Cheraskin, E., Ringsdorf, W. M., Jr., and
Medford, F. H.
**The Eating Habits of High and Low Vita-
min C Users.**
J. Orthomol. Psychiat. 5: #2, 84-88, Second
Quarter 1976.

61. Cheraskin, E., Ringsdorf, W. M., Jr., and
    Medford, F. H.
    The "Ideal" Daily Vitamin C Intake.
    J. Med. Assoc. State Ala 46: #12, 39-40, June
    1977.

62. Cheraskin, E. and Ringsdorf, W. M., Jr.
    Dentists Need More Vitamin C?
    J. Tennessee Dent. Assoc. 57: #4, 177-178, Octo-
    ber 1977.

63. Cheraskin, E., Ringsdorf, W. M., Jr., Medford, F.
    H., and Hicks, B. S.
    **The Relationship of Vitamin C Intake and
    the Total White Cell Count.**
    Nutr. Perspect. 1: #2, 34-36, April 1978.

64. Ringsdorf, W. M., Jr. and Cheraskin, E.
    The Lingual Ascorbic Acid Test.
    Quintessence Internat. 9: #12, 81-85, December
    1978.

65. Cheraskin, E., Ringsdorf, W. M., Jr., Medford, F.
    H., and Hicks, B. S.
    **Relationship of Vitamin C and Skin Symp-
    toms and Signs.**
    J. Canadian Chiroprac. Assn. 22: #3, 97-98,
    October 1978.

66. Ringsdorf, W. M., Jr., Cheraskin, E., and
    Medford, F. H.
    **What Does Vitamin C Have to do with the
    Utilization and Tolerance of Drugs?**
    J. Oral Med. 33: #4, 132-133, October-December
    1978.

67. Ringsdorf, W. M., Jr. and Cheraskin, E.
    The Vitamin C Connection.
    Your Good Health Review & Digest 1: #1, 15-18,
    Premier Issue 1979.

68. Cheraskin, E., Ringsdorf, W. M., Jr., and
    Michael, E. B.
    **The Vitamin C State of a Selected Group
    of Floridian Dentists and Their Staffs.**
    Florida Dent. J. 50: #3, 22-23, Fall 1979.

69. Ringsdorf, W. M., Jr. and Cheraskin, E.
    **Vitamin C and the Metabolism of Analge-
    sic, Anti-Pyretic, and Anti-Inflammatory
    Drugs: A Review.**
    Alabama J. Med. Sci. 16: #3, 217-220, July 1979.

70. Cheraskin, E. and Ringsdorf, W. M., Jr.
    **A Relationship Between Vitamin C Intake
    and Electrocardiography.**
    J. Electrocardiol. 12: #4, 441, 1979.

71. Ringsdorf, W. M., Jr., Cheraskin, E., and
    Medford, F. H.
    Vitamin C and Antibiotics.
    J. Oral Med. 35: #1, 14-17, January-March 1980.

72. Cheraskin, E. and Ringsdorf, W. M., Jr.
    **Vitamin C and Contact Lens Intolerance:
    A Preliminary Report.**
    South J. Optometry 22: #5, 6-8, May 1980.

73. Ringsdorf, W. M., Jr. and Cheraskin, E.
    The Lingual Ascorbic Acid Test.
    1980 Year Book of Dentistry. pp. 284-286.

74. Cheraskin, E.
    **The Name of the Game is the Name: A
    Second and Harder Look.**
    J. Holistic Health. VI: 73-79, 1981.

75. Cheraskin, E. and Ringsdorf, W. M., Jr.
    **Electro-cardiography and Vitamin C: P-
    Wave Height (Lead I).**
    J. Int. Acad. Prevent. Med. 6: #2, 11-20, 1981.

76. Ringsdorf, W. M., Jr. and Cheraskin, E.
Ascorbic Acid and Glaucoma: A Review.
J. Holistic Med. 3: #2, 167-172, Fall/Winter 1981.

77. Ringsdorf, W. M., Jr. and Cheraskin, E.
Vitamin C and Human Wound Healing.
Oral Surg., Oral Med., Oral Path. 53: #3, 231-236,
March 1982.

78. Ringsdorf, W. M., Jr. and Cheraskin, E.
**Vitamin C and Tolerance of Heat and
Cold: Human Evidence.**
J. Orthomol. Psychiatry 11: #2, 128-131, Second
Quarter 1982.

79. Cheraskin, E., Ringsdorf, W. M., Jr., and Sisley,
E. L.
The Vitamin C Connection.
1983. New York, Harper & Row Publishers, Inc.
Paperback, 1984. New York, Bantam Books, Inc.

80. Cheraskin, E.
The Prevalence of Hypovitaminosis C.
JAMA 254: #20, 2894, 22/29 November 1985.

81. Cheraskin, E.
How Common is Vitamin C Deficiency?
J. Alternative Med. 18-19, February 1986.

82. Cheraskin, E.
The "Ideal" Vitamin C Intake.
J. Orthomol. Med. 1: #4, 241, Fourth Quarter
1986.

INDEX

INDEX

A

Alveolar bone loss, 87-93
Appendix, 181-193
Ascorbic acid (see Vitamin C)

B

Bibliography (see Appendix)
Bioflavonoids, 117-120
Blood test (see Plasma ascorbic acid levels)
Bone age, 63-65
Bone loss (see Alveolar bone loss)

C

Cardiovascular, 47-50
Chronologic age, 63-65
Clinical tooth mobility, 79-81, 117-120
Contact lens, 61-62

D

Diet
    dietary vitamin C, 123-127
    protein supplementation, 129-131
    sugar, 133-134

E

Electrocardiogram, 57-60
Epidemiology
    vitamin C, 1-14
    dental school population, 7-8
    dental students, 13-14
    dentists, 9-10
    ordinary working people, 5-6
    orthodontic patients, 11-12
    population groups, 3-4

F

Fatigability, 51

G

General health and disease, 37-71
    bone age, 63-65
    cardiovascular, 47-50
    chronologic age, 63-65
    contact lens, 61-62
    correlations between, 39-41
    electrocardiogram, 57-60
    fatigability, 51
    respiratory findings, 43-46
    skin, 53-55
    vitamin C/general health, 39-41
Gingival hue, 73-76, 113-114, 157-158

H

Health questionnaire, 9-10
Hygiene, 95-97, 99-101, 109-112
Hypovitaminosis C, 3-4

I

Ideal vitamin C state, 161-179
    daily intake, 163-165
    dietary habits, 171-172
    establishment of, 163-165
    human requirements, 173-175
    intradermal range, 167-169
    lingual range, 177-179
Intradermal ascorbic acid test, 19-20
    history, 19-20
    ideal decolorization time, 13-14, 33-35
    method, 19-20
    range, 167-169
    technique used in study, 7-8, 13-14
Introduction, xvi

L

Lingual vitamin C test, 21-22
    correlation of plasma ascorbic acid, 23-25
    decolorization technique used in study, 8, 33-35
    physiologic range, 11-12
    sensitivity following supplementation, 27-28
    technique, 21-22
    test time, 22
    test score range, 177-179

M

Measurement, 15-35
    common way, 17-18
    dietary intake, 33-35
    intradermal, 19-20, 33-35
    lingual, 11-12, 21-22, 23-25, 33-35
    plasma ascorbic acid, 23-25, 33-35
    skin, 29-31
    tongue, 27-28, 29-31
Metabolism, 135-154
    carbohydrate, 145-150
    multivitamin/trace mineral supplementation, 151-
        154
    serum cholesterol, 137-139
    smokers versus non-smokers, 141-144
    tissue levels, 151-154
Multivitamin/trace mineral supplementation, 113-114,
    115-116, 151-154

O

Oral health and disease, 73-120
    alveolar bone loss, 87-93
    blood vitamin C, 79-81, 99-101, 107-108
    clinical tooth mobility, 79-81, 117-120
    gingival hue, 75-76, 113-114
    hygiene, 95-97, 99-101, 109-112
    subclinical scurvy, 77-78
    subclinical tooth mobility, 77-78
    sulcus depth, 83-84, 85-86
    tartar, 103-105, 107-108

Oral health and disease (cont'd.)
    time-release vitamin supplementation, 113-114, 115-
      116
    tissue vitamin C state, 79-81, 85-86, 95-97, 103-105
Orthodontic patients, 11-12, 63-65

P

Plasma ascorbic acid levels, 13-14, 23-25, 33-35, 83-
    84, 99-101, 107-108
Predictive concepts, 155-160
Predictive instrument, 155-160
    cleaning and polishing, 157-158
    gingival response, 157-158
    local therapy, 159-160
    oral response, 159-160
    tissue state, 157-158
Preface: Why this monograph?, xv
Protein supplementation, 129-131

R

Respiratory findings, 43-46

S

Scurvy
    classical, 3-4
    subclinical, 77-78
Serum cholesterol, 137-139
Skin disorders, 53-55
Skin test (see Intradermal ascorbic acid test)
Smoking, 13-14, 141-144
Subclinical tooth mobility, 77-78
Sugar, 133-134
Sulcus depth, 83-84, 85-86, 159-160
Sustained-release supplements (see Time-release)

T

Table of Contents, vii-xi
Time-release multivitamins, 67-71, 113-114, 115-116
Tissue, 8

Tooth Mobility
   clinical, 79-81
   subclinical, 77-78
Tongue, 27-28, 29-31
Tongue test (see Lingual vitamin C test)

V

Vitamin C
   bioflavonoids, 117-120
   blood, 7-8, 79-81
   decolorization time, 14
   dietary, 9-10, 27-28, 123-127
   epidemiology, 1-14
   ideal daily intake, 163-165
   intradermal, 7-8, 13-14, 19-20, 33-35, 167-169
   leukocyte, 3-4
   lingual, 5-6, 7-8, 11-12, 21-22, 23-25, 27-28, 33-35,
      177-179
   measurement, 15-35
   metabolism, 135-154
   nutrition, 12
   predictive instrument, 155-160
   recommended dietary allowance (RDA), 10
   requirements, 173-175
   subclinical, 3-4
   suboptimal, 5-6, 9-10, 11-12
   tissue, 5-6, 8, 27-28, 79-81, 95-97, 103-105

About The Center

Bio-Communications Press is a service of The Olive W. Garvey Center for the Improvement of Human Functioning founded in 1975.

As a non-profit medical, research and educational organization, The Center has been privileged to evaluate patients from all 50 states and 14 foreign countries, conduct clinical and basic research, host 10 International Conferences on Human Functioning and to help stimulate an epidemic of health for the benefit of humankind.

To learn more about The Center, pictured below, send a stamped self-addressed #10 envelope to:

**The Center
3100 N. Hillside
Wichita, Kansas 67219 USA**
316-682-3100

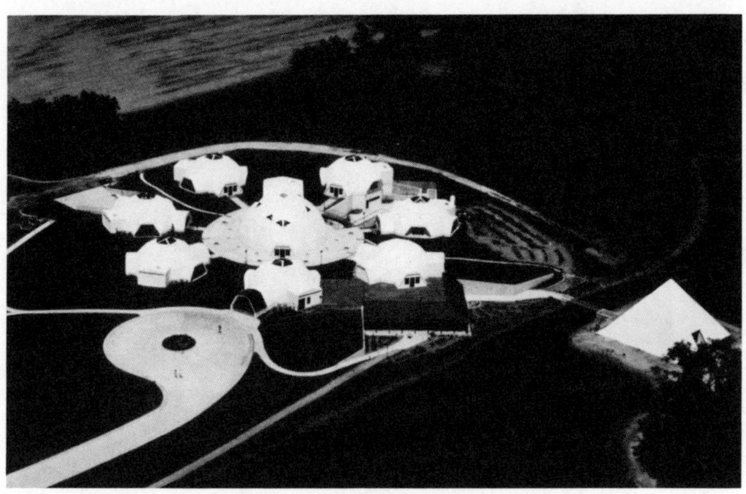

There's More

Bio-Communications Press is publishing a series of books, written by leaders in their fields, to help you stay healthier longer. These are just a few of the books:

The Wonderful World Within You
by Roger J. Williams, Ph.D.
(released in 1987—available now in standard 4-color cover for $14.95 and gold embossed hardcover for $24.95)

The Schizophrenias: Ours to Conquer
by Carl Pfeiffer, M.D., Ph.D., Richard Mailloux, B.S. and Linda Forsythe, B.A.
(will be available in early 1988)

Exploring the Spectrum
by Philip Callahan, Ph.D.

To be among the first to know when these new books become available or to order available books, just fill out and mail the coupon below.

Bio-Communications Press, 3100 N. Hillside, Wichita, Kansas 67219 U.S.A.

☐ Please send me an order form for available books.
☐ Please send me information about upcoming books.

Name _______________________________________

Address _____________________________________

City __________________ State ______________

Country ______________ Zip Code ___________

NOTES

NOTES

NOTES